# Know Your

Please return/renew this item
by the last date shown.

# Know Your
# Complementary
# Therapies

Eileen Inge Herzberg

**AGE** *Concern*

BOOKS

© 2001 Eileen Inge Herzberg

Published by Age Concern England
1268 London Road
London SW16 4ER

First published 2001

Editor   Richenda Milton-Thompson
Production   Vinnette Marshall
Design and typesetting   GreenGate Publishing Services
Printed in Great Britain by Bell & Bain Ltd, Glasgow

A catalogue record for this book is available from the British Library

ISBN 0–86242–309–0

**Bulk orders**
Age Concern England is pleased to offer customised editions of all its titles to UK companies, institutions or other organisations wishing to make a bulk purchase. For further information, please contact the Publishing Department at the address on this page. Tel: 020 8765 7200. Fax: 020 8765 7211. Email: books@ace.org.uk

# Contents

# About the author

Eileen Inge Herzberg has been answering people's questions about complementary medicine for over 20 years. She was the Problem Page Editor for *Here's Health* magazine and founder member of two natural health centres. Her experience of the therapies range from using them for her own health to practising as a massage therapist and healer. She is also a freelance health journalist and has written several books on complementary medicine.

# Acknowledgements

First and foremost I would like to thank Alex Lake for having the good sense to phone an ambulance for me when I was having my heart attack. Also many thanks to the paramedics who gave me first aid and whisked me off to hospital so quickly. And of course, I'll always be grateful to the doctors and nurses at West Cornwall Hospital who probably saved my life.

But I would also like to show my appreciation to the team of healers and therapists who played their part in helping me to recover from my heart attack and heart failure. Special thanks to Faye Moggridge who nursed me back to health (and proof read this book), Rita and Harold Jefferies who held me and healed me when my heart failed me and Olga Statham whose chirpy healing helped so much when I was on what seemed to be a very long road to recovery. I'd also like to thank White Eagle and the Ehama circle – but especially Lu Wray for her healing, friendship and proof reading. I'd also like to say thank you to all the people who sent me absent healing, particularly Cherry Trippe, Angela Enthoven, Beryl Peters, Sashiva O'Donnell, Felicity Bowers and Felicity Kaal Harrison, Elizabeth St John and the other Order of the Ascending Spirit healers.

A very special burst of gratitude to Jesa Macbeth whose teaching, healing, friendship, and 'fairy god-editing' has been an ever present fountain of love and support.

I would never have written *Know Your Complementary Therapies* without Cassandra Lorius (also known as Cassandra Marks). She suggested I write it in the first place, and insisted that I would be well enough to write it at a time when I could barely read, let alone write. She also gave me the perfect homeopathic remedy when I had pneumonia and the antibiotics weren't working.

I'd also like to thank the rest of my support team – Kate Wilson for her brilliant acupuncture and herbs, Bill Watson for his homeopathy, Hira Pascoe for her counselling and psychotherapy, Jean Harris for her healing, Amanda Brown for her yoga, Tim Newman for his zero balancing and Eloha for her special brand of spiritual support. Oh yes, and thank you Alkazar for your extra-ordinary help.

Appreciation also goes to all the therapists and specialists who allowed me to pick their brains – Gopi Warrier for his help with the Ayurvedic section, aromatherapist Julie Eddie and Silvia Baker of the Aromatherapy Organisations Council, naturopath Mark Thompson, herbalist Nikki Green, osteopath Claire Comboye, shiatsu practitioner Val Stagg, psychotherapist Jo May, kinesiologist Richard Beale, astrologer and re-birther Christine Wright, zero balancer Zanna Heighton, nutritionist Amanda Ursell, T'ai chi teacher Felicity Bowers, Alexander Technique teacher Tessa Goldhawk, Bates practitioner Peter Mansfield, Traditional Chinese Medicine practitioners Howard Charman and John Brazier, and general practitioner Dr Geraldine Halls. I'd also like to thank Diane Rush, Jo Ballard, Susan Needham and Marion Green for their contributions to the counselling section. Special thanks to gerontologist Dr Jane Preston who so patiently explained complicated science in terms which were simple enough for me to understand. I'd also like to thank Dr Helen Dziemidko, Margot Pinder at the Foundation for Integrated Medicine, columnist Katherine Whitehorn and author/musician Richard Wentk.

Thank you also to Lucy and Elsie, the two Apple computers who helped me write the book, Barnes Cook who looked after them and Peggy Rickerby who generously gave me Elsie when Lucy was stolen. I'm also grateful to Truro, Penzance and Age Concern England reference libraries – where would I have been without them?

On the production side, thank you to Tam for her typing of the lost manuscript when Lucy got kidnapped, Richard Holloway and Vinnette Marshall at Age Concern England, and Richenda Milton-Thompson for her patient and sympathetic editing.

# Introduction

Welcome to *Know Your Complementary Therapies*. I hope that you enjoy reading it as much as I enjoyed researching and writing it. It is aimed mainly at older people who have never tried complementary therapies and want to know more before they try them. But I hope too that people who already use complementary medicines will find the book interesting and helpful.

As I was writing *Know Your Complementary Therapies*, I was struck by just how rapidly interest in complementary medicine was growing – and how popular it had already become. For example, a House of Lords Select Committee Report on Complementary and Alternative Medicine, carried out in 2000, found the following trends in the UK:

- Sales of herbs, homeopathic remedies and aromatherapy essential oils had soared by 50 per cent to £93 million between 1993 and 1998. They could rise to £126m by 2002.
- As a nation, we spend about £1.6 billion a year on complementary and alternative medicine.
- Five million patients a year consult a complementary practitioner.
- There are 60,000 complementary practitioners to choose from.

*Know Your Complementary Therapies* is divided into three main sections. Section One describes what complementary medicine is, how it differs from ordinary medicine and how it can help with the ageing process. Section Two describes the different therapies and answers the questions you are most likely to ask. Section Three advises you how to choose the best therapies and therapists to meet your particular needs, and where to go for help.

I hope that I have answered the questions that you are most likely to ask. For example, I thought you might be interested in whether or not acupuncture hurts, or whether you need to believe in healing for it to work. (Incidentally, the quick answer to both of these questions is 'no', but see the relevant sections of the book for more detailed answers.)

Although I have been involved in complementary medicine since 1981, I still learned a great deal when I was researching the book. I hope that you will have fun reading *Know Your Complementary Therapies* regardless of whether you have plenty of personal experience or whether you are thinking of trying them for the first time.

Enjoy!

Eileen Herzberg

2001

# SECTION 1

# 1

# What is Complementary Medicine?

This book is about that other sort of medicine – the sort that does not rely on man-made drugs or surgery. Some people call it natural medicine, some call it complementary or alternative, and some have started to call it CAM (Complementary and Alternative Medicine). This chapter outlines its history and describes what the various labels mean.

## *History*

Ever since humans first walked the earth we have tried to make sense of ourselves and the world around us. Through trial and error we found out about plants and trees – from the best wood to burn on the fire to the dock leaves growing conveniently close to the stinging nettles. Keeping warm was just as important to our health as easing incidental aches and pains. When someone was ill, loved ones would pray for their recovery – but then it was all too obvious that whether someone lived or died was in the hands of powers that were greater than human.

In a confusing world when many women died in childbirth and babies often didn't live long enough for childhood let alone adulthood, we had more questions than answers.

Over 5,000 years ago we looked to the natural world for clues and the Chinese developed a system of medicine which was based on observation of themselves and the world around them. Traditional Chinese medicine considers the world of nature and humankind in terms of energy – yin and yang – contracting and expanding.

In India over 7,000 years ago, the ancient seers or wise ones took to the hills and meditated on the essence of life and found answers which encompass every aspect of life including meditation, prayer, exercise and what we eat and drink. Their findings about the basic elements of life were passed down by word of mouth until 1000BC when they were written down in the Vedas, the divine Hindu book of knowledge which became the foundation for Ayurvedic medicine.

The Western world also had a form of natural, holistic medicine which was concerned with the basic elements of life. It dates back to ancient Greece, when the great philosopher and doctor Hippocrates made some astute observations which formed the foundation of Western medicine. He trained in Egypt, so much of what he says may be based on ancient Egyptian medicine.

Hippocrates thought people could be understood and treated according to their temperaments and body types, and that these in turn could be related to the four elements of fire, water, air and earth. We are all made up of these four elements and good health was based on keeping them all in balance. These elements were seen as the basic building blocks for life and they are absent when we die. We lose our body heat, we stop breathing, we dehydrate and return to the earth.

## The elements related to health and illness

The idea that the basic elements, including fire, water, earth and air, are essential to understanding health and illness seems to be universal.

**Ancient Greeks**: fire, water, earth and air

**Traditional Chinese medicine**: fire, water, earth, metal (air) and wood, the element of growth

**Ayurvedic medicine**: fire, water, earth, air, and space or ether, the spiritual dimension

Although Hippocrates lived in the fifth century BC, he still has a profound influence on modern medicine. For example, doctors still take the Hippocratic oath, in which they promise to cause no harm to their patients.

Hippocrates also described other concepts which are still in use today:

- **Nutrition** 'Let food be thy medicine and thy medicine thy food.'
- **Massage** 'The physician should be experienced in many things but assuredly in rubbing, for rubbing can bind a joint that is too loose and loosen a joint that is too tight.'
- **Spiritual healing** 'The heat which oozes out of the hand, on being applied to the sick is highly salutary.'
- **Germ theory** 'By contact, some diseases may be communicated from one to another.'

At the time of the ancient Greeks, people believed that our lives and deaths could be explained by the actions of gods and goddesses. Careful note was taken of dreams, for these were messages from the gods. Illness was also seen as a divine message and priests and priestesses were in charge of healing.

Looking at the life cycles of plants and animals and the movement of the sun and the stars, we understood that we were part of a natural cycle of birth, growth, decay, death and rebirth just as the sun was reborn each morning and died each night.

With the spread of Christianity, the Church became the central point of learning and medicine. Spirituality and healing were still part of the same process, but we didn't understand how our bodies worked. This started to change after the first authorised public dissection of a human body took place in France in 1375.

The established Church view of the world was turned on its head by Copernicus who, in the early 16th century, suggested that the sun, not the earth, was the centre of the universe. This was backed up by Galileo who invented the telescope around a century later. The observations of Sir Isaac Newton and that apple falling to the ground resulted in more than just an understanding of gravity. The separation of religion from science had begun. But it was the philosopher René Descartes who completely turned established thinking on its head.

Descartes thought – and enabled others to think – in a completely new way. Because of this, we were no longer tied to the idea that all events were determined by divine intervention:

- He **separated mind from body** in his famous phrase 'I think, therefore I am'. **Logical, rational thought** started its ascendancy.
- He suggested that the best way to study the body was to divide it up into as many pieces as possible. This is known as the **reductionist** approach.

These ideas formed the basis of modern Western medicine and it led to a much greater understanding of how our bodies work and how we are affected by the world around us. We also learned about the medicinal properties of poisons such as arsenic and sulphur, and operations became increasingly dramatic and dangerous.

## Pioneers of thought

Nicolaus Copernicus 1473–1543
Galileo Galilei 1564–1642
René Descartes 1596–1650
Sir Isaac Newton 1642–1727

Pioneers of natural medicine such as Samuel Hahnemann (who developed homeopathy) were so disturbed by the poisoning and blood letting associated with scientific medicine that they looked for gentler ways of helping people. In fact natural medicine as we know it today is partly old, traditional medicine which has been in continuous use for centuries, and partly relatively new forms of medicine which have been developed over the past 200 years.

Natural medicine is also known by many other names:

- Alternative medicine
- Complementary medicine
- Integrated medicine
- Traditional medicine
- Holistic medicine
- Energy medicine

## Alternative medicine

'Alternative medicine' was the buzzword when natural therapists wanted to offer something that was completely different from conventional medicine. People who were in favour of natural medicine wanted to be seen to be different. The phrase alternative medicine is still used as a way of differentiating natural medicine from modern medicine. But there is a slightly militant edge to the word 'alternative'. It demands that people make a choice between drugs and surgery and more natural forms of treatment – it is no longer fashionable to be alternative.

## Complementary medicine

As natural therapies became more accepted by doctors and the NHS, the term 'complementary medicine' began to be used. This marked a recognition of the fact that natural medicine and orthodox medicine were not competing against each other, but could be used to complement each other. For example, a person may decide to take anti-inflammatory tablets as well as have osteopathy for rheumatism, or use the homeopathic remedy arnica to speed healing after an operation.

## Integrated medicine

The term 'integrated medicine' is relatively new and points the way to a future where there is no separation between different forms of medicine. In China, they already have a form of integrated medicine as the hospitals and doctors choose the most appropriate form of treatment, irrespective of whether it is drugs or herbs, anaesthesia or acupuncture, operations or manipulation — or indeed a combination of different methods.

British medicine is moving towards a more integrated approach. In 1999, the Foundation for Integrated Medicine and the Guild of Health Writers made an award for Good Practice in Integrated Healthcare and there were 80 entries. One of the finalists was Glastonbury Health Centre Complementary Medicine Service. Here a conventional GP's surgery also offers herbal medicine, homeopathy, massage therapy and osteopathy for the price of an NHS prescription.

But this is the most public face of integrated medicine. Advances are also happening in much more subtle ways and have been so successful that the original, 'alternative' therapy has become invisible. Biofeedback is perhaps the best example of this. Biofeedback uses instruments which tell us what is going on inside our bodies, so that we can change it. It started off as an unconventional idea which helped people learn how to relax, meditate and do healing work. Today, it is used in physiotherapy departments in hospitals to control pain, blood pressure and urinary incontinence. In fact, by the nature of their work physiotherapists use a lot of natural medicine techniques. They are trained in massage and manipulation, and many now use acupuncture.

Nurses are also starting to use natural medicine as they recognise its benefits, both for themselves and for their patients. Like physiotherapy, nursing lends itself to natural therapies. For example, nurses already have physical contact with their patients, and it is just a short step to add therapeutic touch (a form of healing) or massage. In fact massage used to be a standard part of nurse training at the beginning of the 20th century and re-introducing a more "hands on" approach is helping nurses to reclaim their original skills and increase job satisfaction.

Counselling and psychotherapy used to be thought of as part of alternative medicine; now they are so mainstream that they are not included in many surveys of complementary medicine. A survey of fundholding GP surgeries in England and Wales carried out by the Mental Health Foundation in 1997, found that 40 per cent of these employed a counsellor and about 28 million counselling treatments were carried out each year. If anything, the number has grown since the introduction of Primary Care Groups and Trusts. It is certainly a popular form of treatment, and can almost be described as mainstream. It is 'complementary' in the sense that it complements other forms of treatment and does not use drugs or surgery.

Perhaps one day we will not talk about alternative, complementary or even integrated medicine – they will all be part of a holistic system of medicine. But for now at least, alternative, complementary and integrated medicine all refer to natural medicines and the ways in which they relate to modern medicine.

## Perspectives on 'integrated medicine'

At the moment, if you mention integrated medicine to your GP, they may assume that you are talking about moves to integrate hospitals, GPs surgeries and community care within the NHS. Instead of reducing healthcare into different sections, the NHS is making important steps towards a more holistic approach by trying to provide 'seamless care'. Indeed, the new National Service Framework for Older People argues for patient-centred care, in which different professionals work together as a team, so the patient gets the best possible treatment.

## *Traditional medicine*

The term 'traditional medicine' is a way of describing any form of natural medicine that has been around for a long time – these are the therapies which have a long history behind them. Examples of traditional medicine include traditional Chinese medicine, Ayurvedic medicine and traditional herbal medicine. Dietary therapy, which is concerned with what we eat can also be described as a form of traditional therapy, but nutritional therapy which is concerned with both food and vitamins and minerals is relatively new. Therapies such as reflexology, kinesiology and zero balancing are also relative newcomers.

Examples of traditional medicine include:

- Traditional Chinese medicine
- Ayurvedic medicine
- Traditional herbal medicine
- Dietary therapy
- Naturopathy.

## *Holistic medicine*

> 'The curing of the part should not be attempted without treatment of the whole'.
>
> Plato, 3rd century BC

> 'to see a world in a grain of sand
> and Heaven in a wild flower.
> Hold infinity in the palm of your hand
> and eternity in an hour'.
>
> William Blake (1757–1827) *Auguries of Innocence*

As the name implies, 'holistic medicine' means medicine for the whole person – that is healing for body, mind and spirit. There are many different ways of looking at holism; it is not confined to natural medicine as it describes an overall approach to health and disease, rather than a particular form of therapy.

The holistic approach is becoming increasingly important within the NHS. For example, the NHS standards of care for cardiac rehabilitation (as outlined in the National Service Framework for Coronary Heart Disease) state that before patients are discharged from hospital their 'physical, psychological and social needs' should be assessed.

It doesn't matter whether you are seeing an ordinary doctor or a natural health therapist – some have a holistic approach and others do not. For example, if you go to a doctor with backache, you may simply be given painkillers. A holistic doctor may ask some additional questions and discover that you are also depressed and feel that you do not have enough support in your life. This may result in your being referred for counselling. Similarly, some natural health practitioners have a broad, holistic approach, while others will just be interested in your symptoms.

Holistic practitioners are concerned about the 'whole person', and as such they are interested in every aspect of your well-being and how these all interrelate.

## Body – the physical aspect of your being

This includes your physical symptoms, but it is also concerned with how you are affected by your environment. For example, are your aches and pains made worse because you sleep in an uncomfortable bed, or sit in an uncomfortable chair? Do you eat enough or too much? Could you be eating something that is causing the problem?

Almost any holistic doctor or practitioner will probably ask these kind of commonsense questions.

## Mind

Concern for the health of your mind does not only involve looking at your mental symptoms, but also at how you are affected by the world around you. For example, if you find it hard to concentrate, this may be caused by all sorts of things, from bereavement to stress.

## Emotions

How you feel at the moment can be affected by what has happened in the past and what you anticipate may happen in the future. Your joy and sadness, hopes and fears can have a big impact on how well you feel.

## Spirit

A holistic practitioner will also be concerned about your spiritual life and at least be aware that it will affect your physical and mental well-being. For example, you may be tossing and turning at night because your spirit is uneasy if you are feeling guilty about something that you have done or not done. Or you may be wrestling with important questions such as the meaning of life and death.

Body, mind, emotions and spirit are all inter-related. For example:

- Your **backache** may be caused by bad **posture** (body).
- The **posture** may be caused by the way you feel about yourself (**emotions**) – when we are **depressed** or feel over-burdened, we tend to slump and throw our backs out of proper alignment.
- The **depression** might be caused by false beliefs (**mind**) about others not caring about us or because we believe we cannot have, or do something we think is really important to us.

- Because we are depressed, we may also feel that life has lost its **spiritual meaning** and joy.

It can be a vicious circle. But it can be turned into a virtuous circle if we were to practice simply standing up straight and taking deep breaths from time to time. This may help us feel better both physically and emotionally, and we can help that process along by looking at the attitudes we may have had that led us to slump in the first place. It is the inter-relatedness of body, mind, emotions and spirit that is important.

Holistic medicine isn't just what doctors and therapists do, it is also the way that they do it. For example, a doctor who explains what he or she is doing while taking your blood pressure and puts you at ease, is taking your blood pressure in a holistic way, paying attention to your emotions as well as to your physical complaints.

Some therapies such as homeopathy, acupuncture and Ayurvedic medicine, are holistic by their very nature, and the questions may be very probing as this helps the doctor or therapist decide on the best form of treatment. For example, you may be asked whether you like fatty food, or if you have any food cravings, or whether you feel better or worse for exercise, even whether you prefer sleeping on your right side or the left. Your answers will help the practitioner to decide on the most appropriate form of treatment.

But even holistic therapies can be used in non-holistic ways. Not all practitioners have been trained to think holistically, and this can make it difficult for them to see the whole picture. On the other hand, holism may not be appropriate in the circumstances. For example, if you fall over and bruise yourself, the homeopathic remedy arnica will be helpful – regardless of what is happening emotionally or spiritually. The arnica may also help with the shock of the accident, but that is incidental. For first aid and emergencies, it is better to act first, and think holistically afterwards.

## Popular therapies

More and more people are using complementary and alternative medicine – the recent Institute of Complementary Medicine poll on behalf of the BBC suggested that one in five Britons are now opting for such therapies.

(ICM poll on behalf of the BBC, August 1999. Source: Foundation for Integrated Medicine evidence to the House of Lords, Science and Technology Committee III, Complementary and Alternative Medicine – CAM.)

## *Examples of holistic medicine*

Any form of medicine can be holistic – what is important is the way it is practised.

One of the principles of holism is that everything affects everything else. In natural medicine, some therapies rely on the holistic theory that if you hurt or cure one part, it has an effect on your whole being. Examples of holistic medicine include:

- **Traditional Chinese medicine diagnosis** By looking at your tongue and feeling your pulse, a practitioner can tell what is happening throughout your whole body.
- **Acupuncture** Putting a needle in one part of the body can have an effect on other areas. Auricular acupuncture (ear acupuncture) uses points in the ear to affect the whole body.
- **Iridology** By looking at your eye, an iridologist can tell what is happening to your whole body, what has happened in the past and what may happen in the future.
- **Reflexology** This is based on the idea that what happens in your feet mirrors the rest of your body.
- **Visualisation and relaxation techniques** are based on the idea that what happens in your mind affects your body, and what happens to your body affects your mind.

## Energy medicine

These are therapies which address your life force — the animating force that is uniquely you and is no longer there when you die.

### The life force

The Chinese call this 'chi', 'jing' and 'shen'
Indians call it 'prana'
Homeopaths call it 'the vital force'
Healers call it 'energy' or 'life force'

We all recognise what it feels like to have no energy, to feel emotionally and physically flat. Our get up and go has got up and gone! Energy medicine helps us to recharge our batteries.

Energy is also known as:

- Power
- Force
- Vigour
- Vitality.

The therapist works with our own energy, helping us to help ourselves by balancing our natural healing energy and giving it support. The focus is not on trying to match the illness with a medicine or a therapy, but rather on our own ability to heal ourselves. However, energy therapy is not just concerned with our own energy, the therapies themselves work with energy.

- Homeopathic remedies contain energy – it is not the medicine that makes us feel better, it is the **energy in the medicine** that makes us feel better.
- In spiritual healing, it is **divine or universal energy** that makes us feel better.
- Acupuncture unblocks **our own energy channels**, helping us to receive divine or universal energy.

Energy medicine is a dance between our own ability to heal ourselves, the power of the treatment or medicine we are using and a guiding force which is responsible for all healing. Examples of energy medicine include:

- Homeopathy
- Bach flower remedies
- Acupuncture
- Healing

## Do-it-yourself natural therapies

Apart from seeing a complementary medicine practitioner, you may also want to do something to help yourself. Examples of therapies that can be approached in this way include:

- Yoga
- T'ai chi
- Chi gong
- Alexander Technique
- Meditation

But of course, all forms of complementary medicine are concerned with you – you are where all the treatments begin and end. This reminds me of a joke I saw on a greetings card. A doctor says to a patient: 'I like your tie … Your hair looks really nice … That jacket really suits you'. The caption reads: 'Complimentary medicine'!

# 2

# How Complementary Medicine can help with the Ageing Process

Complementary therapists view ageing as a natural process. It is as natural as breathing in and out. If we live long enough, grey hair and other signs of ageing will be inevitable in humans, just as trees get wider and more gnarled with age.

As we get older, how healthy we are will partly depend on:

- What we start with.
- What we do with ourselves.
- What happens to us during our lives.
- How we react to what happens to us.

## What we start with

The health we are born with is the starting point. Complementary therapists call this core state of health our **constitutional health**. It will depend partly on the health of our parents and partly on our own unique characteristics. In Chinese medicine it is known as 'jing', or 'ancestral chi'. In scientific terms, this is the level of health that is determined by our genes.

### CHOOSE YOUR PARENTS CAREFULLY

If our parents lived long, healthy lives, there is a good chance that we will do the same. When a baby is born, we can see how the baby has 'her mother's eyes' or 'his father's nose' or some other physical family characteristic. We are just as likely to inherit tendencies towards particular types of ailments. Every family has its Achilles heel, a part of the body that tends to be weaker than the rest or a tendency to suffer from some diseases more than others. For some families, it may be a predisposition towards heart disease, for others it may be cancer. These are tendencies, not predictions. They form part of the pattern of health that we are born with.

Complementary medicine is concerned with preserving your core level of health.

## WHAT WE DO WITH OURSELVES

'If I'd known I was gonna live this long, I'd have taken better care of myself.' Eubie Blake (1883–1983) in *The Daily Telegraph* Quote of the Day, 13th February 1983.

Even if we are born with iron strong constitutions, we can expect to suffer the consequences in old age if we don't look after ourselves.

Different complementary therapies have different views on how to live a long and healthy life, but they all agree that doing anything to excess will affect our health. We all know that smoking is bad for us and over-eating is bad for us. The Chinese say that if we want to live long, healthy lives, women should not have too many children and men should not ejaculate. The theory is that men lose energy when they release their sperm. In India, tantric yoga also teaches men to control their sexual energy and bring it up into the higher 'chakras' or energy centres rather than releasing it in the normal way.

Everything we do influences our health in one way or another. This is one of the reasons why complementary health practitioners ask so many questions. They need to know what we do, in order to see the important patterns in our lives.

The questions therapists ask are likely to cover the following range of topics:

- What we eat
- Our home life
- Our work life
- Families
- Our leisure activities
- Our spiritual lives

- Our level of exercise
- What sports activities we participate in
- Our love affairs and marriages
- Whether we are workaholic or lazy.

## What happens to us

This can be a natural consequence of what we do, or it can appear to be totally outside of our control. It may include the following:

- The consequences of births, deaths and marriages
- The consequences of not having children or being married
- Relationships and their consequences
- Viral and bacterial diseases
- Accidents and injuries
- Obesity and malnutrition.

The main reason we now live longer is that, thanks to better hygiene and nutrition, fewer women and babies die in childbirth and we are less likely to die from viral and bacterial diseases. However, we are now more likely to suffer from stress and die from cancer or heart disease.

We must have learned something about how to deal with diseases that come from outside ourselves. Now we are trying to understand diseases which come from within: why our cells lose their sense of identity and become cancers, why our blood vessels clog up and cause disease and why we have all sorts of diseases which can be blamed loosely on stress.

### HOW WE REACT TO WHAT HAPPENS TO US

If, like me, you have ever experienced walking on fire, you'll know what it feels like to feel totally in control of yourself and your sur-roundings. I knew the fire would not burn me – and it didn't. For those few moments it felt as if I was able to move without friction, without being affected by the world around me.

Unfortunately, I have not found out how to treat ordinary life like this. I can see that, theoretically at least, it should be possible to go through life without being hurt by what it has to throw at me. But I haven't yet acquired the knack.

In fact we are designed to deal with life's difficulties and this natural ability is known as 'homeostasis'. It comes from the Greek words homoios meaning similar and stasis, meaning standing – homeostasis is our ability to stay the same by automatically adjusting to change. For example, we adjust to hot weather by sweating. As the sweat evaporates it draws out the heat of the body, which has a cooling effect.

In many different ways, complementary medicine is concerned with homeostasis, supporting your own natural ability to cope with what life throws at you. For example, if you have been involved in a car accident, after the hospital doctors have put you back together again and mended your broken bones:

- An **osteopath** or **chiropractor** will help you deal with the physical aftermath by realigning your joints.
- A **counsellor** may help you deal with the emotional consequences by helping you come to terms with the facts of the situation.
- A **healer** may help your energy body recover from the shock, making it possible for your energy body and your physical body to be re-united.

The different therapies have a single aim – to help you to recover from the accident so that you can get back to where you were before it happened.

Complementary medicine also helps us keep our balance through the more everyday ups and downs of life and this is where therapies such as T'ai chi, Chi gong, yoga and meditation can be helpful. Complementary medicine also recognises that our own reaction to events can have a significant impact on our health.

## The power of positive thinking

Dr Steven Greer, psycho-social oncologist and researcher at the Royal Marsden Hospital found that 80 per cent of women with breast cancer with 'fighting spirit' were still alive after 10 years, and after 15 years, 45 per cent were still alive (45 per cent died of other causes). But only 17 per cent of women who stoically accepted the diagnosis or who felt helpless in the face of their cancer survived 15 years. Six out of seven similar studies have shown that people with cancer who have a positive attitude have a higher survival rate than those who are hopeless.

(Source: Bristol Cancer Help Centre, The Question of Hope Conference, 1995)

### TICKING CLOCK THEORY

Scientists also see ageing as a natural process, like a clock ticking away from the moment of conception. Scientists recognise that it is just as natural for the body to grow old as it is for the baby to grow into a child and onwards into maturity. It is similar to what happens to annual plants which die once the flowers have turned into seed heads. The Pacific salmon is similarly programmed to die after reproduction.

Humans are much more complex than flowers or fish and the ageing process is not so obviously linked to reproduction, but ageing may also be controlled by hormones. Some researchers think that the hormone dehyudroepiandrosterone (DHEA) holds the key to human ageing. It is found in higher levels among younger people and experiments have shown that DHEA supplements help laboratory rats live longer.

The human growth hormone may also be involved in human ageing as we produce less of it as we get older. The growth hormone is responsible for looking after our tissues, particularly muscle tissues. Young people with a growth hormone deficiency tend to be small and have weak muscles. In older people, reduced growth hormone levels are one of the reasons for the skin becoming thinner and muscles weaker.

While scientific medicine is still searching for the clock and the hormones which are responsible for ageing, traditional Chinese medicine (TCM) has had the answer for centuries. The TCM view is that we are all born with a certain amount of jing, or ancestral chi, which is mainly stored in the kidneys (see the section on 'Traditional Chinese medicine' in Chapter 4).

## WEAR AND TEAR

Scientific medicine recognises that life is a delicate balance between the forces of destruction and repair. Destructive forces leading to cell death are balanced by the forces that repair this damage. The scientific view is that there is a limit to how long we can carry on repairing and maintaining each cell for the following reasons.

- Damage tends to accumulate with age

With complementary medicine, the aim is not just to attend to the current problem, but to heal past traumas and illnesses. For example, someone who has been cured of asthma, may then find that skin symptoms return and it is the turn of their old eczema symptoms to be treated. It is almost as if complementary medicine can turn the clock backwards.

- The body gradually loses its capacity to repair the damage

Complementary medicine can support the body's ability to repair damage in a number of ways. It can do this by providing the energy and nutrients the body needs to repair itself. It can also do this by helping the body to work as smoothly as possible, in order to minimise wear and tear. For example Andrew Still, the founder of osteopathy, compared the human body to a machine. He believed that if the machine were serviced regularly, and kept in the best possible condition, wear and tear would be minimised.

Traditional medicine and energy medicine do this more subtly by keeping our energy bodies well balanced (see Chapter 6, 'Energy Medicine', for more information on energy bodies).

## THE DRYING OUT PROCESS – GLYCOSYLATION, CROSS LINKING

Wrinkled skin, stiffening of the joints and many of the symptoms we associate with ageing are caused partly by a chemical reaction in the body. This is where proteins and sugar (usually glucose) link together and become rigid. This process is known as 'cross linking' or 'glycosylation'.

When foods such as meat or bread are heated, the proteins combine with sugar and turn brown in a process known as caramelisation. In our bodies, the sticky by-product of this chemical reaction can literally gum up our cells. In human cells, cross linking happens when two protein molecules link together – usually with the help of a sugar bridge. This stiffens the molecules and will affect us in different ways, depending on where the proteins are. For example, when the collagen protein in skin links together, the skin loses its elasticity and we get wrinkles.

Collagen is also present in ligaments and muscles, so it is not just our imagination, joints and muscles really do become stiffer as we get older as a result of cross linking. The cells in the muscles can become so tightly linked that the texture changes and becomes more like a ligament than a muscle and the ligaments become so stiff, they become almost like bones. This cross linking process also accounts for:

- Some forms of heart disease where the arteries become less flexible, less able to move blood around the body (sometimes known as hardening of the arteries).
- Some forms of diabetes where the blood vessels in the pancreas can stiffen to such an extent that it is no longer able to make insulin.
- Cataracts and other eye problems where cells are no longer able to line up to let the light through and the eye becomes opaque.

Cross linking happens spontaneously, even in test-tubes, and it seems to be an inevitable part of ageing. Complementary therapies can offer ways of helping us make the best possible use of the healthy cells, the cells that haven't cross-linked. Many complementary therapists recommend diets which are low in protein and sugar – the raw ingredients behind this cross linking process.

### FREE RADICAL DAMAGE

Free radicals are the body's bullies. They can cut other molecules down the middle, chop pieces off them, link them to another molecule (contributing to cross linking) and can cause cancer and cell death.

Free radicals can damage DNA (deoxyribonucleic acid – the 'genetic coding material' or reproduction instructions within each cell). This causes mutation that can lead to cancer. Also, if the free radicals attack cell membranes, which are mainly composed of fat, they can produce a similar effect to fat turning rancid in the sun. The cell membrane loses its ability to contain the contents of the cell and, if it is not repaired quickly, this can result in cell death.

The older we get, the more free radical damage accumulates. This may explain why the following diseases become more common as we get older:

- Arthritis
- Short term memory loss
- Dementia
- Parkinson's disease
- Alzheimer's disease
- Cancer
- Strokes
- Heart disease where cholesterol has built up in the blood vessels.

But free radicals are a natural by-product of the way we use oxygen – so we also have natural ways of making sure that they don't get out of hand. We do this with the help of certain enzymes which are known as 'free radical scavengers' and 'anti-oxidants'. We make our own free radical scavengers from enzymes with exotic names like SOD (superoxide dismutase), from anti-oxidants such as vitamins A, C and E, and from amino acids which come from the foods we eat.

We cannot stop free radicals from being created because we need oxygen, but we can keep them in check with the help of free radical scavengers, anti-oxidants and amino acids. No wonder practically every anti-ageing book you turn to extols the virtues of a healthy diet and vitamin supplements. Complementary therapies also keep free radicals under control by supporting the body's immune system and some therapists recommend the use of fasting and other methods of giving the body a good clean out.

## SLOWING DOWN

Our cells can only divide and grow a limited number of times (see the box on the Hayflick limit overleaf). The fewer divisions that are left in a cell's life, the more slowly the cell divides.

The slow-down in the ability of cells to divide and grow means that it takes longer for cuts to heal. This is one of the reasons why skin becomes more fragile and prone to ulcers as we get older.

Another effect of this slow-down is that it becomes more difficult for the body to protect itself against infection. Our white blood cells and all the other cells in our immune system need to divide and grow very quickly to fight infection – and this gets increasingly difficult as we age.

In addition, the slow-down of these processes of cell division and growth means that cancer becomes more common. The cells in our immune system are responsible for removing damaged and mutant cells before they become cancers. Therefore, this slow-down means that they may give mutant cells the time needed to become cancers. This may explain some of the age-related cancers such as cancer of the prostate and colon.

Complementary medicine cannot stop the slow-down in the cells' ability to divide and grow completely, but it can support the immune system and give it the physical and energetic nourishment it needs.

## Cell division: the Hayflick limit

In 1961 Leonard Hayflick discovered that there is only a limited number of times that a single cell can reproduce itself. He found that when normal human cells are in a culture, they go through a finite number of cell divisions and then stop. This is known as 'the Hayflick limit'.

Hayflick found that normal cells reproduce themselves about 100 times if they are taken from foetal tissue, but if they are taken from a 70 year old they reach their limit of ageing after 20 or 30 divisions. The older the tissues, the fewer times the cells divide. Some cells are able to reproduce themselves more often than others.

The Hayflick limit does not apply to the division of all cells – eggs and sperm cells continue to divide, which is why children can live longer than their parents! Unfortunately it also seems that cancer cells do not have a limit to the number of times they can reproduce themselves. Bone, joint, muscle and nerve cells cannot divide to replace themselves, so they are particularly precious.

## CHIPS OFF THE DNA BLOCK

Every time a cell divides, a bit gets chipped off the DNA and the chromosomes get shorter and lose control of what happens in the cell. Scientists are not sure how this affects our health, although there are several theories. It may play a part in atherosclerosis (the build up of plaque on artery walls which is associated with heart disease) and the slow-down in the body's ability to heal wounds and fight infection. Again, there is nothing that complementary medicine can do to stop this process from happening completely, but it may slow it down and can help the unaffected cells to work at peak efficiency.

# Age-related diseases

As we have seen, as we get older, so do our cells. It is part of being human. Doctors often say 'it's your age' which is both irritating and unhelpful, but it is also true that some diseases occur more often in older people. A list of common, age-related complaints is given in the box.

## Age-related complaints

Almost everyone will experience some deterioration in both their eyesight and their hearing.

- **Osteoarthritis** is the type of arthritis that is caused by wear and tear of the joints and is the most common form of arthritis in the over 65s. It affects nearly half of all people over 65 and most people over 70 have some arthritis in their joints.
- **Osteoporosis** is where bones become smaller and more fragile and more likely to break. It is about four times more common in women than men, particularly after the menopause. About one in four women over 65 will develop osteoporosis.

- **Diabetes** (late onset or type 2 diabetes) is where the pancreas cannot produce enough insulin to control blood sugar levels. Symptoms include extreme thirst and passing a lot of urine. About one in every five people in the 65–74 year old age group are likely to have diabetes.
- **Bladder incontinence** is also increasingly common as we get older.
- **Cancer** is one of the top three killers. About half of all cancers occur in people over 65. More people suffer from lung cancer than any other cancer, but your chances of having lung cancer are significantly reduced if you do not smoke.
- **Heart disease** is the leading cause of death for people over 65, accounting for 45 per cent of all deaths. Again, you are much less likely to suffer from heart disease if you do not smoke.
- **Strokes** are caused by a sudden disturbance in the blood supply to the brain (cerebrovascular disease) which accounts for 9 per cent of deaths among the over 65s. One stroke in three leads to immediate death, and another one in three causes permanent disability such as paralysis (often on one side of the body) or loss of speech.
- **Transient ischaemic attacks (TIAs)** occur when there is a brief interruption of the blood supply to part of the brain, resulting in temporary loss of vision, speech, sensation or movement. It only lasts for minutes, or at the most a few hours. If it lasts for 24 hours, it is called a stroke.

Because the cells in the brain cannot reproduce themselves, there seems to be a link between **Parkinson's disease, Alzheimer's disease** and various forms of **dementia** and ageing.

- **Parkinson's disease** is caused by a breakdown in the nervous system and symptoms include tremors or shaking of the head and hands, leading to progressive loss of muscle control and the ability to walk. There may also be dementia and depression. It is not until a brain area has lost 70–80 per cent of its cells that Parkinson's disease symptoms occur. People may not notice anything at all unusual until at least half of the area has been lost.

- **Alzheimer's disease** is clearly age related since the risk of suffering from it rises dramatically in old age: Alzheimer's disease affects 0.5 per cent of 65–70 year olds and 1.5 per cent of 70–75 year olds. The incidence reaches a maximum of 30–35 per cent in 90 year olds. Up to 50 per cent of the brain cells have already been lost by the time the symptoms of Alzheimer's disease are bad enough to need help. Alzheimer's disease is a form of dementia which includes memory loss and personality changes. It accounts for about half of all dementias.
- **Other dementias** – about 20 per cent of dementias are caused by problems with the veins. A build up of cholesterol in the walls of the arteries and veins reduces the flow of blood to the brain and can cause dementia and other problems.
- **Mini-strokes** – where a small blood clot damages the brain – can also cause dementia.

## A healthy old age

The extraordinary thing about the diseases and ailments associated with ageing is that we can have them without suffering from them. Post mortems often reveal diseases that the individual was blissfully unaware of. For example, over half the people with Alzheimer's disease are only discovered as a result of post mortem examinations, as they are symptom free.

Unexplained clumps inside the cells which are similar to the clumps associated with Parkinson's disease have been discovered in people who have no symptoms at all. Post mortems can also reveal heart disease and cancers, even though the person wasn't aware of having any problems. Doctors often see apparently normal joints which are giving people extreme amounts of pain, yet other people's x-rays may show considerable damage and distortion even though the person is relatively free from pain.

Our aches and pains may be due to diseases – or they may not. Feelings of well-being may be due to freedom from disease – or they may not. While modern medicine focuses on finding cures for what goes wrong, complementary medicine is more concerned with what goes right. Although different forms of complementary medicine vary in their approach to disease, they share a common basic belief in the body's ability to heal itself. What complementary medicine does is to give our innate healing ability a little help.

Complementary medicine also recognises the fact that there is a certain mystery behind health and disease. It is a complicated process which can be affected by everything we do. For example, a study reported in the United States journal *Demography* and quoted in the July/August 2000 issue of *Healthy* found that people who go to church live longer than those who don't. According to this piece of research, non-churchgoers die on average at 75, while weekly churchgoers live an extra seven years. It is hard to tell exactly why this should be: it could be that they are less likely to smoke, or they may have a better social life – or it could have something to do with the power of prayer and the fact that they have a more active spiritual life.

## THE IMPORTANCE OF HORMONES

Hormones have a crucial part to play in the ageing process of the body. Children with **hypogonadism** remain physically forever young because the glands don't develop properly. Boys do not produce the testosterone they need to grow into physical manhood and girls do not develop the oestrogen necessary for puberty and ovulation. At the other end of the spectrum, **progeria** causes people to age at such a rapid rate that a 19 year old may have the appearance of a person of 65.

## LONG LIFE

Theoretically, we can all live to be 120 – this is how long individual cells and tissues can survive. This upper estimate is what nature has given us, and so far at least, it has not been changed by medical science. But more of us do seem be living longer.

In 1955, the Queen sent 302 Happy Birthday telegrams to people who had reached 100 or more. Ten of them were 105 or over.

Telegrams do not exist any more, so the Queen sends cards instead. In 1999, she sent 3,542 Happy 100th Birthday Cards, and another 391 cards to people who were 105 or over.

# Long livers

Luigi Cornaro, a Venetian nobleman wrote *A Treatise of Health and Long Life* and lived to be nearly 100. He believed in a low calorie diet, regular sleep, exercise and the enjoyment of leisure time.

Sir Winston Churchill lived to be 90 and he drank a quart of brandy, smoked ten cigars a day and never ate anything but rare beef. (*Superyoung* by Dr David Weeks and Jamie James, Hodder & Stoughton, 1998)

The Bristlecone pine trees, found in California, are the most ancient beings in the world. Some of these trees are more than 4,500 years old, with no end in sight. (*Ageing Concepts and Controversies* by Harry R. Moody, Pine Forge Press, 1998)

At the beginning of the 21st century, more of us are living longer thanks largely to better nutrition which has meant that fewer women die in childbirth, more babies and children survive into adulthood and fewer people die from infections.

# Life expectancy

The average life expectancy at the beginning of the last century was 46–50
Girls born in 1998 can expect to live till they are 80
Boys born in 1998 can expect to live till they are 75

Source: *International Brief Gender and Aging, Mortality and Health* by Kevin Kinsella and Yvonne J. Gist, International Programs Center, US Department of Commerce Economics and Statistics Administration Bureau of the Census, October 1998.

In 1880 out of every million babies born, only 161,164 would have lived to be over 75; now it is nearer 613,000.

Source: *Time of Our Lives* by Tom Kirkwood, published by Phoenix and quoted by Katherine Whitehorn in *Saga Magazine*.

Only 25 per cent of what we call ageing may be caused by the physical consequences of getting older, the other 75 per cent of ageing is sociogenic according to ageing expert Dr Alex Comfort. Sociogenic means that it is caused by the social 'rôle' which our folklore, prejudices and misconceptions impose on 'the old'. In other words, only 25 per cent of ageing symptoms are outside our control. We have some choice about the rest if we shake off our prejudices.

(For more information about this aspect of ageing, see *Listening to Midlife – turning your crisis into a quest*, by Mark Gerzon, Shambala, 1996, and the chapter on 'Aging: Real and Imaginary' in *New Old: Struggling for Decent Ageing* by Ronald Gross *et al.*, Anchor, 1978).

# 3

# What is the Difference between Complementary Medicine and Modern Medicine?

One way of thinking about the difference between the two forms of medicine is to consider gardening. A gardener who follows the complementary medicine approach uses natural organic techniques such as companion planting to keep away black fly, and sand or broken eggshells to protect delicate plants from slugs. On the other hand a gardener who uses a modern medicine approach sprays with insecticides and puts out slug pellets.

While scientific medicine focuses on cures for diseases, complementary medicine is concerned with helping us to heal ourselves. Complementary medicine is helpful when our own natural resources need support in coping with the challenges and stresses of life. Modern Western medicine is helpful when our natural resources have broken down.

People who practice complementary medicine have many different ideas and philosophies, but they share a common basic belief — that we can all heal ourselves, we just need a little help from time to time.

Complementary medicine sees symptoms as signs that the body is actively involved in healing itself and may need support in the process. For example Samuel Thomson, one of the founders of modern herbal medicine, thought that high temperatures should be encouraged because they were the body's way of fighting infection. At the same time the conventional approach to fevers was that a high temperature was a potentially dangerous state; the main aim of medicine at the time was to bring the temperature down.

Thomson revived the ancient herbal tradition which saw fever as the body's way of generating heat to fight off the invasion of cold disease. Far from being a danger signal, he saw a high temperature as something that should be encouraged, since it showed that the body was doing what it could to fight off the disease. His ideas were partially based on the ancient Indian healing sweat lodges where patients sweated out their toxins in a tent which was heated with very hot stones, a bit like a sauna. Thomson also recommended that fevers should be treated with cayenne pepper (capsicum minimum) which also raises the body temperature.

The emphasis with complementary medicine is on health, and what can be done to make the person more healthy. 'Health' can be described in many different ways, for example as:

- Positive feelings of well-being.
- Feelings of happiness, joy.
- Freedom – the ability to do what you want in life without being limited by ill health.
- Absence of disease and pain.
- The ability to bounce back to health after a trauma. To recover full health as quickly as possible after accidents, infections and emotional stress.
- Feeling fulfilled and content with one's life.

Most of us are not completely healthy because we carry the effects of different traumatic events that have happened in our lives. Many forms of complementary medicine are concerned with healing the original trauma as well as the continuing symptoms. For example, osteopaths are not just concerned with making your current aches and pains go away, they also treat the source of the problem – which may be an accident that happened many years ago. This emphasis on health means that complementary medicine is interested in people rather than disease. People are unpredictable and with any form of medicine or treatment some will benefit, some will get worse, and some may be unaffected. What do the people who get better have in common? How can we recognise the people who are likely to benefit in the future? These are the kind of questions which interest complementary medicine practitioners.

Because of this emphasis on individuals' ability to heal themselves, complementary medicine practitioners specialise in particular forms of treatment rather than in different parts of the body or types of disease. One of the effects of this is that two people with the same complaint may be given very different treatments, because it is the people who are treated not the disease. For example, if you go to an acupuncturist requesting treatment for your arthritis, the practitioner will feel your pulse and look at your tongue, try to understand what is happening and then decide on the best way of treating you. Even though two people may both be suffering from arthritis, because they are individuals they will need to have needles sited in different places (see the section on 'Acupuncture' in Chapter 6). This is one of the reasons why it is so difficult to research complementary medicine in the conventional way.  People, rather than complaints, are being treated, so it is hard to have controlled trials where the treatment has to be consistent.

Complementary medicine practitioners use natural medicines, but all forms of medicine are natural – even 'man-made' medicines have to start with natural ingredients. Some medicines even come from the same plant, but are prepared and prescribed differently. Take foxglove, or to give its official Latin title, Digitalis. Digitalis is the name of a herb which is used by herbalists for people with heart problems. Digitalis is also the name of a homeopathic remedy that is used for people with heart problems. It is known as Digoxin when it is used in modern medicine for people with heart failure. The foxglove is prepared differently, depending on whether it is for a pharmaceutical company, a herbalist or a homeopath.

- For the pharmaceutical preparation, only the **active ingredients** of the foxglove are used.
- For the herb, the **actual plant** is used.
- For the homeopathic remedy, the **energy** of the plant is used.

## *Complementary practitioners*

When you see a complementary practitioner, you may notice some differences between them and your ordinary NHS GP or hospital doctor. Perhaps the biggest difference is time. Expect to see your complementary practitioner for at least 30 minutes to an hour. You may also notice some more subtle differences when you see a complementary practitioner which may be a result of their training and general background.

Training for complementary practitioners varies widely depending on which form of complementary medicine the practitioner is learning. They don't dissect bodies, although they may become very familiar with skeletons. Depending on which therapy is being taught, a large part of their training will be concerned with emotional issues as well as physical symptoms. Complementary medicine students often practice on each other so that they experience the therapy they are learning about. This means they know what it feels like to be on the receiving end of their treatment!

Complementary medicine students and practitioners see fewer people than NHS doctors do. This means that they don't have as much experience of seeing hundreds of different people all suffering from the same complaint; but it also means that they don't suffer from so much stress, with the pressure of dealing with everyone as quickly as possible.

At the moment, most complementary health practitioners work in private practice and can set their own fees. This is changing: the NHS is starting to buy in services from complementary health practitioners, but this process is quite new. Most complementary practitioners work in:

- Complementary health centres
- Natural health centres
- Therapy rooms
- Beauty salons

There are also self-help therapies such as yoga and T'ai chi which may be held almost anywhere including village halls, gyms, and dance studios.

## HEALTHFOOD SHOPS

Healthfood shops often sell natural medicines. Some of the people who work in healthfood shops know a great deal about natural medicine. They often work in healthfood shops because they believe in the products that are sold and can be a good wonderful source of information about which products are best for different complaints. They may also know a great deal about the practitioners in the area, and which ones might be best to consult for particular problems.

## NATURAL HEALTH CENTRES/COMPLEMENTARY HEALTH CENTRES/THERAPY ROOMS

There is usually a more leisurely atmosphere and fewer patients per practitioner in therapy rooms, complementary or natural health centres than in ordinary GPs' surgeries. Most of the people who practice complementary medicine are part of the private sector. So if you see a complementary health practitioner, he or she is unlikely to be part of the NHS – although this is changing. This means that you will probably have to pay for treatment, and you will see the practitioner for half an hour to an hour or more.

# Where to use complementary medicine – and where to use modern medicine

Complementary medicine is helpful when our own natural resources need support in coping with the challenges and stresses of life. Modern Western medicine is helpful when our natural resources have broken down.

Modern Western medicine can be traced to the Greeks in the fourth century BC when there were two main schools of medicine. One school was founded by Hippocrates, who believed that the whole individual needed to be studied and treated for good health. The other school was founded in the town of Knidos, and its followers concentrated on looking at disease as an invader that had to be destroyed and medical intervention was aimed at directly relieving the symptoms of disease.

## EMERGENCY

There are times when disease does literally strike like an invader – and has to be dealt with accordingly. Serious, life threatening events which come out of the blue include:

- Pneumonia
- Heart attacks
- Broken bones
- Damage following an accident
- Appendicitis.

These should be dealt with immediately with Knidos style medical intervention. In just such situations, heroic action is needed and modern, Western medicine comes into its own.

Theoretically, complementary medicine could also be helpful in life threatening situations, but complementary practitioners do not normally work in accident and emergency departments, or even visit patients when they are ill in bed. This means that they do not have the experience to cope with emergency situations.

## BREAKDOWNS

Heroic, modern Western medicine is also needed when parts of our bodies break down. Modern medicine can provide mechanical, spare part surgery, for example:

- Hip replacements
- Joint replacements
- Heart transplants
- Heart surgery (replacement valves, pacemakers etc)
- Kidney transplants
- Cataract operations
- Setting broken bones
- Surgery for cancer
- Surgery for benign lumps.

When our bodies no longer function properly, modern medicine can provide life-saving substances such as:

- **Insulin** when the pancreas can no longer make its own.
- **Thyroxine** when the thyroid can no longer make its own.

- **Oxygen** when the lungs, heart or blood have problems in providing enough oxygen on their own.

## DIAGNOSIS

Always see your GP for a conventional diagnosis. GPs can refer you for blood and urine tests and set up x-rays and scans. It is very important that you are diagnosed accurately, so that you know what's wrong with you mechanically.

An accurate diagnosis can help you choose what form of treatment to use. For example, if that cough is just a cough, you may want to try natural ways of treating it. But if it is pneumonia, this is potentially such a serious problem that it should be treated with antibiotics, although you may also want to have treatment from a homeopath, acupuncturist or healer to mobilise your own self-healing mechanism.

## THE LIMITS OF MODERN MEDICINE

Medical students in Australia are told the following story to help them understand the limitations of modern medicine.

An elderly woman was dying in hospital. Her relatives were called around her bedside and the priest was brought in to give the last rites. Because she had had so many different things wrong with her for a long time, she had been taking lots of different tablets. As she was dying, all medication was stopped, she had such a short time left that they even stopped giving her painkillers. She lived through the night, and after a day or two, she started to get better and went on to live for several years in excellent health.

This story is told to medical students because it shows, firstly, that no-one really knows whether someone is going to live or die. Secondly, it is told because it shows that medicine can sometimes do more harm than good. Obviously you shouldn't stop taking medicine that has been prescribed for you – but it is advisable to question whether any of your symptoms are actually being caused by the medicine that you are taking.

Anything can cause problems, no matter how innocent it may appear. I say that from experience. After I had a heart attack I was told to take aspirin to prevent another one. I suffered from diarrhoea for months after the heart attack and had all sorts of tests and scans, but it wasn't until I was suffering from internal bleeding that one of the doctors suggested I stop taking the aspirin. The result was miraculous! My diarrhoea stopped and my recovery started.

## Side-effects

Side-effects are such an accepted part of modern medicine that there is even a name for them – **iatrogenic disease**. About 20 per cent of hospital admissions are caused by iatrogenic disease.

(Source: *The Health of Adult Britain*, 1841–1994. Edited by John Charlton and Mike Murphy, Office for National Statistics, Stationery Office.)

Obviously the most natural form of medicine is no medicine at all, but there are times when our own healing mechanism needs support. This is where complementary medicine comes into its own. As we get older, we are more likely to need some form of support to help us stay in the best possible health.

### PREVENTION

Prevention is better than cure. Legend has it that in ancient times the rich, influential Chinese paid a fee to be kept healthy – they didn't pay when they were sick.

Prevention is becoming an increasingly important part of modern medicine as doctors realise the importance of diet, exercise and healthy living. But there are also many forms of natural medicine to choose from to help you to stay as healthy as possible.

Health is not just an absence of pain and disease, it is a positive feeling of well-being, so whatever you do to improve your health, you will know if you're on the right track if you enjoy the therapy itself, or if it makes you feel happier in some way.

You can relieve stress with relaxing therapies such as:

- Massage
- Healing
- Reflexology
- Zero balancing.

You could also consider self-help therapies such as:

- T'ai chi
- Meditation
- Yoga.

Take the advice of nutritional and dietary therapists, and keep your energy in balance with treatment from a healer, an acupuncturist or a homeopath. Take care of your emotional health by having counselling to put your mind at ease.

## Western medicine and complementary medicine

- Always take the medicine that has been prescribed for you
- Ask your doctor or complementary health practitioner about what you are taking
- If you are taking medicine from your GP, it is very important to tell him or her about any natural medicines you are taking
- If you are taking a remedy from a complementary medicine practitioner, it is also important to tell him or her about any medicine you are taking from your GP

**Questions to ask:**

- Can my symptoms be related to what I am already taking – can these symptoms be side-effects?
- What is this for and how will I know if it's working?
- Is it compatible with the other medication and natural remedies I am taking?
- Am I taking the lowest dose that is likely to have an effect?

The effects that medicines have on us change as we get older because they stay in our bodies for longer as the kidneys and liver get less efficient.

If you have been on medication for many years, it is a good idea to check with your doctor to see whether you still need so much.

## MYSTERY ILLNESSES

Although modern medicine has very sophisticated equipment and techniques for diagnosis, sometimes our aches and pains defy analysis. Here is a short list of some complaints which may have a medical explanation or may not.

- Vague aches and pains
- Vague stomach upsets
- Feeling tired all the time
- Little or no energy
- Headaches.

The ability to cope with vague, unusual symptoms is one of the basic differences between modern medicine and complementary medicine. Complementary medicine, particularly energy-based medicine, is usually more concerned with helping your own healing mechanism cure whatever the problem is, so a concrete diagnosis is not always necessary.

## LONG TERM CHRONIC COMPLAINTS

If you have had a problem for some time, complementary medicine may be helpful, particularly where modern medicine has not worked.

## CONVALESCENCE

Complementary medicine can also be helpful if you are recovering from an illness or accident. For example, complementary medicine can play an important rôle during the recovery period after a heart attack and most doctors recognise the value of relaxation, diet and gentle exercise at this time.

## LIMITATIONS OF COMPLEMENTARY MEDICINE

Time is a major limitation. Complementary medicine works by supporting the body's own healing mechanism, and this can take time to work. In an emergency, for example, there simply may not be enough time to allow the natural remedies to work, even if they were available. Natural medicines are not always slow to take effect, but you may not know which is the best medicine to take and finding out can take valuable time.

Further limitation may be imposed by lack of availability and experience. Complementary medicine practitioners tend to work ordinary office hours, by appointment, and may not be available if there is an emergency. Unlike your GP, they do not have to offer 24-hour care. Also, most complementary medicine practitioners work in private practice and tend to focus their attention on chronic complaints, and so they have less experience of emergency medicine than their colleagues who work in NHS hospitals.

There are also natural limits to complementary medicine. It cannot mend parts of the body that are broken. It can only help the body to repair itself or to adjust to difficult situations. For example, complementary medicine cannot help you grow a new hip, but it can help you to make the most of the hip you've got.

## LIMITATIONS OF MODERN MEDICINE

'Mystery ailments' can confound modern Western medicine. If there is a problem that cannot be diagnosed by tests and scans, it will be hard to treat. Similarly, modern medicine often proves useless when confronted with immune system breakdowns as it cannot restart or improve the immune system.

In addition, modern medicine can cause side-effects.

## *Death and dying*

One of the biggest differences between complementary medicine and modern medicine is in their approach to death and dying. There comes a point when it is clear that a person has reached the end of their life and there is nothing that any form of medicine can do, except to make the transition as comfortable and painless as possible.

At this stage, modern medicine can call on painkilling drugs such as morphine which has a numbing effect not only on the physical pain, but also on the mind and the emotions. Side-effects such as difficulty in breathing may also be caused by morphine. It takes great skill and experience to judge what is needed in these situations.

Perhaps it is because doctors and nurses have recognised the limitations of drugs in terminal illness that complementary medicine has come to play an increasingly important role in the hospice movement. Although different branches of complementary medicine have different philosophies, many view the whole process of dying as just that – a process. It is as important a part of life as birth, indeed it is very similar. In fact, it could be argued that we need midwives to help us through both transitions.

In the 1970s, Dr Elisabeth Kübler-Ross conducted some interesting research into near death experiences. This is where the heart stops beating and for all intents and purposes the person has died, but is then revived. Dr Kübler-Ross interviewed thousands of people who had had a near death experience and found remarkable similarities in all their stories:

- They said that they looked down on their body and saw the people who were trying to save their lives.
- They said that they went through a dark tunnel and could see a very bright light at the other end.
- There were people they knew and loved, such as parents and spouses, who were ready to greet them, but they were told to go back because it wasn't the right time.
- They experienced feelings of overwhelming love.
- They said that when they 'came back' their lives had changed forever and they were no longer afraid of death.

Scientists tend to think that this can all be explained away as an hallucination caused by lack of oxygen. This may be so. But equally, it may be a glimpse of what really happens when we die. As far as complementary medicine is concerned, it doesn't matter whether this is true or false. What does matter is that people die as 'well' as they can be in body, mind and spirit.

There are many ways in which complementary medicine can help with the **physical difficulties** of the dying process, and in a sense, dying is no different from any other chronic complaint. The role of complementary medicine is to support the body's own healing process, even where the next stage in the process may be death.

Our **state of mind** is always important and the things that need to be done to put the mind at rest are the same, regardless of whether the challenge is to live or die. It is particularly important to resolve long-standing conflicts and feelings of guilt, and to tie up unfinished business. Counselling and healing can be particularly helpful.

**Emotions** are also very important, and complementary medicine in the form of aromatherapy or healing for example, can have a very valuable, soothing part to play in the dying process.

**Spiritually,** dying is obviously a particularly significant time and visits from a priest or spiritual healer can be helpful.

Because dying is a process that involves moving from one state of being to another, it takes a certain amount of **energy.** This is where some of the energy-based medicines such as homeopathy, acupuncture or healing can be very useful.

## PAIN RELIEF

The way that modern medicine tackles pain relief is mainly through drugs which are known to have pain-relieving qualities. They usually work in a way which is similar to the way a key opens a lock. For example, morphine is designed to fit into a part of the brain that is normally activated by endorphins, the body's natural form of pain relief. Drug-based pain relief can be very effective, particularly if the dose is accurately judged so that there is enough pain relief to dull the pain, but not so much that it dulls the senses.

The disadvantage of drug-based therapy is that it can dull other senses along with the pain. This can affect people in several different ways. For example, it can:

- Make breathing more difficult.
- Make thinking more difficult.
- Reduce appetite.

- Cause constipation.
- Make it more difficult to eliminate liquids.

The advantage of using natural medicine for pain relief is that it does not create these side-effects. The disadvantage is that it may not be readily available. Natural forms of pain relief can certainly be as effective as drugs. Take acupuncture for example: this can be such a powerful form of pain relief that operations can be done using only acupuncture as an anaesthetic.

# SECTION 2

# 4
# Traditional Medicine

## Introduction

Everyone wants to live a long and healthy life – so it is not surprising that the quest for the magic elixir for immortality is common to most cultures.

In China, thousands of years ago, the shamans took to the hills to try to discover nature's secrets. Their hard won knowledge filtered down to the valleys and was finally written down in manuscripts 3,500 years ago. The Chinese believe that we are born with a certain amount of energy which needs to be carefully preserved if we are to live a long and healthy life.

In India, the wise ones took to the mountains, the highest mountains in the world. Their approach was to rise above their bodies, to transcend the physical world, and focus on the spiritual world. In order to do this, they trained the physical body so that it could act as a strong vessel for the spiritual body.

In Britain, wise women (healers or 'witches') were persecuted, and it is hard to find a continuous tradition of natural medicine. Alchemists, who tried to turn base metal into gold in their search for the elixir of youth, tended to be recluses, so the idea never became mainstream. The nearest we have to their tradition today is transpersonal psychology, which turns the base metal of dreams into golden insights. Britain's oldest medicine is probably herbal medicine – but the only form of medicine which covers such broad areas as the Indian or Chinese traditions is naturopathic medicine which is only a century old in its present form.

The complementary therapies in this section are all complete systems of medicine in that they have something to offer our body, mind and spirit. You may be more familiar with the different parts of these traditional medicines than you are with the complete system. Yoga for example, is part of Ayurvedic medicine, so is meditation. Acupuncture is part of traditional Chinese medicine, so is T'ai chi. Wholefood diets and fasting are part of naturopathic medicine, so is hydrotherapy.

Traditional medicine encompasses a range of different therapies, but each traditional system includes the following:

- Diet
- Fasting and cleansing
- Exercise
- Herbal medicine
- Massage and/or manipulation

The main reason why traditional medicine is not widely known in Britain is that there are not that many practitioners. There are only around 310 qualified practitioners of naturopathic medicine in the UK at present, and a mere 60 qualified practitioners of Ayurvedic medicine. This may change – partly because of the growing interest in complementary therapies, and partly because of increased training facilities.

# Traditional Chinese medicine

'Traditional Chinese medicine' is a blanket term which covers all the different therapies that have been traditionally used in China.

## History of traditional Chinese medicine (TCM)

TCM goes back about 5,000 years, to the shamans, medicine men and mountain recluses who lived off a sparse, herbal diet. In their quest for long life, they developed exercises and breathing techniques and practised martial arts such as kung fu. They believed that the mists of the mountains were rich in the special force or energy known as chi (pronounced chee).

By 1500 BC, references to herbal medicine were being made on oracle bones. The wild men from the mountains started to come down into the markets to display their kung fu skills and trade their herbs and plants for tools, cloth and wine. They eventually settled in the villages, but many centuries later, at a time of great turmoil, the 'xian' or 'immortals' took to the mountains again. This time, the quest was for the elixir of everlasting life.

Medicine was shrouded in mystery and magic, in fact the symbol for medicine was 'wu', which also meant sorcery. In 1122 BC the bottom part of the character was changed to the symbol which meant wine and the character changed to 'yi' or doctor. The link between medicine and wine was important as alcohol had many properties which made the medicine more effective.

The legendary emperor Shen Non who lived around 3494 BC is thought to be the father of Chinese medicine and agriculture, but it wasn't for another 2,000 years that anything he said was written down. He is credited with discovering the idea of yin and yang (see the box on page 54). Chinese medicine became a profession during the Han dynasty, around 206–222 AD, when the first medical textbooks were written.

## The five elements in Chinese medicine

- **Earth** – stomach and spleen meridians
- **Metal** – lung and large intestine meridians
- **Water** – bladder and kidney meridians
- **Wood** – gallbladder and liver meridians
- **Fire** – heart and small intestine meridians

Over the centuries TCM developed into a complete system of medicine, despite various attempts to suppress it. In 1929 for example, doctors returning from training in Western medicine in Japan wanted to ban all forms of non-Western medicine. There was a huge outcry against the idea and a delegation of doctors pleaded with the Nationalist Government in Nanjing to keep traditional forms of medicine. They succeeded, and March 17 became known as 'Chinese Doctors Day'.

There has been a vast amount of research into the effectiveness of TCM and, in China today, TCM and Western medicine are practised alongside each other. In 1983, for example, public health officials in Beijing announced that a 400 year old prescription for the treatment of haemorrhoids (piles) had proved to be 96 per cent effective and was officially designated as a cure. The cure consisted of 'an injection of insect secretions on sumac leaves mixed with crystal salt'.

Acupuncture came to Britain in the 19th century, but it has only been in the past 50 years that TCM has been taught as a complete system of medicine. During the last two decades, British acupuncturists have begun taking extra training to learn about Chinese herbal medicine.

## What happens when you have a consultation?

When you first meet your practitioner, he or she will ask you a lot of questions about your medical history as well as about your current health problems and general lifestyle. The questions will cover a wide range of topics including your eating and sleeping habits, the time of day you feel most active, and what makes your complaint better or worse. The practitioner will look at your tongue and feel your pulse in order to find out which aspects of your energy are out of balance and in what way, before deciding on the best treatment for your problem.

### Balancing the energy flow

TCM uses many different techniques to balance the energy flow in the body including:

| | |
|---|---|
| **Cupping** | A glass is placed over an acupuncture point which draws blood to the surface. This is used to ease painful conditions such as arthritis. TCM students learn cupping before they are taught any of the other treatments. |
| **Moxibustion** | A burning herb (mugwort) is placed on an acupuncture point via an acupuncture needle, but it can also be placed on a slice of ginger or garlic. |

**Point injections** Vitamins are injected into particular points. This is rarely used in Britain.

The main TCM treatments which are used in Britain include:

**Acupuncture** See the section on 'Acupuncture' in Chapter 6.

**Chi gong** See the section on 'Chi gong' in Chapter 9.

**Herbs** Apart from plants and flowers, Chinese herbs include snakes, minerals, gallstones from cow or water buffalo, fungus, even 'dragon bones' (made from crushed, fossilised bones). The herbs themselves come in many forms; dried pieces that need to be boiled up, powders, granules, pills and liquids.

**Diet** The TCM view of food is that it can be used as medicine. The Chinese have much more sophisticated versions of Jewish chicken soup, which is known to cure all ailments! These include, for example, salted fish heads with tofu and ginger for fevers and palpitations; lotus root, daikon radish or watercress soup in pork broth for chest infections and colds (see the section on Dietary therapy in Chapter 8). Like Ayurvedic medicine, TCM is also concerned about the way you eat and its effect on your health. Eat slowly, chew well, focus your attention on eating (not on television) and do not eat when you are emotionally upset.

**Tui'na** This means 'push pull' and consists of various physical techniques including acupressure, massage and manipulation. Tui'na is based on the idea that we experience pain when blood and energy stagnate. It releases trapped blood and energy so that they flow freely. The therapist will

> work on points which are close to the pain as well as some which seem far away from the pain to encourage the movement of energy through the whole energy channel (meridian). The therapist also works on particular points which are related to particular problems. For example, if you have eye problems such as cataracts, eye pain, night blindness, itchy eyes, one sided headaches, or have knee pain, the therapist may treat Gallbladder 37 – also known as 'bright light'.

## What is TCM suitable for?

Because traditional Chinese medicine is a complete system of medicine which focuses on improving health rather than fighting disease, it can be used for anything and everything. For the purposes of this book, however, we will look specifically at conditions which are common in older people. TCM is particularly useful for treating arthritis, low energy, heart disease and backache.

### ADVANTAGES OF THIS FORM OF TREATMENT

- You will be given advice and guidance about your general lifestyle from what you eat, to how you exercise.
- Some of the treatments such as tui'na are very enjoyable.

### DISADVANTAGES OF THIS FORM OF TREATMENT

- You may be asked to change your lifestyle, your diet or your exercise pattern as part of the treatment.
- You may not like the idea of some of the treatments, such as acupuncture.

### SELF-TREATMENT

TCM is not suitable for self-treatment. You need to see a TCM practitioner who can diagnose where your energy is out of balance, then advise you accordingly about the best things you can do to help yourself, such as practising Chi gong exercises or changing your diet.

# Theory of ageing

According to traditional Chinese medicine, the ageing process is governed by three forms of energy:

- Pre-heaven essence or **jing**
- Post-heaven essence or **chi**
- **Kidney essence.**

### PRE-HEAVEN ESSENCE OR JING

This is the energy we inherit from our parents at the moment of conception. It determines what we look like, our basic constitution, strength and vitality. It is the amount of energy we are born with and although it gets depleted by everyday living, we cannot make new jing. The best we can do is to conserve what we are born with.

The best ways of conserving jing is to try and lead a balanced life: to keep a balance between work and play and to eat a well-balanced diet. Men should not have too much sex – and when they do have sex they should try not to release sperm. Women should not have too many children.

Breathing exercises, T'ai chi and Chi gong also conserve jing.

Provided we lead reasonably well-balanced lives with enough rest, exercise and nourishment, most of us have enough jing to last 100 years or more.

### POST-HEAVEN ESSENCE OR CHI

This is the essence we do have some control over, as it is extracted from food and fluids all through our lives. It is created by having a good diet and a healthy lifestyle.

### KIDNEY ESSENCE

This is a mixture of pre-heaven essence and post-heaven essence. Kidney essence controls growth, reproduction, development and maturity. It also controls the various stages of life: birth, puberty, menopause and death.

Ageing is due to the decline of kidney essence. If the kidney essence is flourishing and abundant the kidneys are strong and there will be great vitality, sexual power and fertility. If kidney essence is weak, the kidneys are weak and there will be lack of vitality, infertility or sexual weakness. Kidney essence decreases as you get older, and this weakens the kidneys and the energy associated with the kidneys. Symptoms associated with weak kidney energy include:

- Poor memory
- Weak bones
- Poor concentration
- Dizziness
- Bad back
- Weak knees and ankles
- Weak teeth
- Poor bladder function
- Incontinence
- Breathlessness
- Deafness
- Falling hair
- Grey hair
- Lack of will power
- Tendency to become easily discouraged
- Lack of vitality
- Tiredness.

Kidney energy holds the key to ageing, but it also controls wisdom. According to traditional Chinese medicine, as jing declines, wisdom increases.

# Yin and yang

Traditional Chinese medicine views life in general, and the body in particular, as a balance between two natural forces: yin and yang.

Each force has its own particular quality and will create different symptoms when it is out of balance.

For example:

- Yang is male, active and stimulating and represents light, heat, dryness and contraction.
- Too much yang may cause sudden pain, inflammation, spasms, headaches and high blood pressure.
- Yin is female, passive and tranquil and represents darkness, coldness, moisture and swelling.
- Too much yin may cause dull aches and pains, chilliness, fluid retention, discharges and tiredness.

# Ayurvedic medicine

The word Ayurveda comes from two Sanskrit words: 'ayur' meaning life and 'veda' meaning knowledge. It is an all-embracing system of medicine which draws together all aspects of life and relates them to health and well-being. Treatments include herbs, meditation, yoga and dietary therapies.

## *History of Ayurvedic medicine*

Ayurvedic medicine has its roots in the Hindu religion and is over 7,000 years old, the oldest medical system in the world. It all began when the wise ones (rishis or seers) meditated on the essence of life – and were given some very detailed answers. Their discoveries formed the basis of 'Ayurveda' which was passed down by word of mouth from generation to generation, until it was written down in 1000 BC. Today's Ayurvedic doctors use a shorter version of this text, which dates back to 1000 AD. It is the most popular form of medicine in India where Ayurvedic doctors work with Western doctors.

Ayurvedic medicine came to Britain with Indian immigrants in the 1950s and 1960s, and at first it was barely heard of outside the Indian community. Meditation and yoga were the first aspects of Ayurveda to reach a wider public, and more recently oiling and massage have became fashionable stress reduction treatments. It is only in the past few years that the complete Ayurvedic medical treatment has started to become better known in Britain.

Two new developments will increase the popularity of Ayurvedic medicine in Britain:

- The first Ayurvedic degree course outside India started at Thames Valley University in 2000.
- The first free Ayurvedic hospital outside India opened in London in 2000.

## What happens when you have a consultation?

The practitioner will ask you questions about your health – both past and present. He or she will also be interested in your lifestyle and may ask you quite detailed questions about your diet, what you do to relax, your working life, your social life, and your family life. You will also be given a physical examination which will include feeling your pulse, and examining your tongue, urine and stools. The practitioner will also notice your eyes, skin, nails, even the quality of your voice and your general appearance.

The aim of this part of the consultation is to decide on:

- Your basic constitution
- How it came out of balance
- The appropriate treatment.

## Your constitution

In Ayurvedic medicine, your constitution is the key to your pattern of health – this is known as the **dosha**. There are three doshas: vata, pitta and kapha.

We are all born with a dominant dosha, sometimes we are born with a mixture of two, equally dominant, doshas. Our dosha determines who we are and includes such features as our hair colour, body shape, the foods we crave, and the type of illness which we are most likely to get. We change as we get older, tending to be more kapha when we are young, pitta when we are adult and vata when we are old.

## THE DOSHAS

### Vata

Vata is like air or wind, constantly on the move, it controls the central nervous system. Vata people tend to be:

- Thin
- Overactive
- Easily exhausted
- Chilly
- Unlikely to sweat
- Emotionally erratic
- Fearful, anxious, insecure
- Creative, and full of ideas.

Vata imbalance can be caused by irregular meals, too little sleep, a promiscuous sex life, outbursts of anger and jealousy and any form of over-exertion.

- **Avoid** lentils, beans, peas, leeks, coffee and spinach.
- **Eat** eggs, milk, oats, almonds and basmati rice.

Vata people are prone to joint pains, rheumatism, mania and depression.

### Pitta

Pitta controls the digestive system and all biochemical processes. Pitta people tend to be:

- Of medium build
- Full of stamina
- Warm
- Sweaty
- Steady with few mood swings
- Judgmental when they are angry
- Intellectual and ambitious
- Good at carrying things through.

Pitta imbalance is often triggered by indigestion, alcohol abuse and feelings of grief or fear.

- **Avoid** sesame oil, pepper, garlic, lemons, yoghurt, chillies and alcohol.
- **Eat** apples, avocado, cabbage, spinach, wheat and chicken.

Pitta people are prone to ulcers, gastritis, cystitis and urinary tract infections.

## Kapha

Kapha governs the balance of tissue fluid controlling cell growth and the firmness of the body. Kapha people tend to be:

- Fat or heavily built
- Lazy but with good stamina
- Cold
- Sweaty
- Greedy and possessive, but calm and caring
- Slow thinkers, but can organise well.

Kapha imbalance can result from a lack of physical exercise, sleeping during the day and the effects of the seasons.

- **Avoid** butter, chocolate, milk, sugar, avocado, bananas and meat.
- **Eat** broccoli, apples, tomatoes, onions, chillies, peppers and spices.

Kapha people tend to suffer from chest problems, asthma, bronchitis, colds and sinus problems. They can also suffer from depression.

### DIFFERENT WAYS OF LOSING YOUR BALANCE

In Ayurveda, good health comes from all three forces being in harmony, with none of the doshas being too strong or too weak. Illness comes from one or more of these forces being out of balance. The source of the problem will have a big influence on the kind of treatment which will be recommended.

## Accidents or injuries

This will include any kind of blow, cut, sting, bite or physical accident. Treatment will be first aid or surgery.

## Physical, internal illnesses

These may include tumours, inflammations and blockages. Treatment will be a combination of medicine, diet and yoga.

## Mental and emotional triggers

Anger, fear, hatred, laziness, misery and pride can also disrupt balance. Treatment will involve counselling and meditation.

## Natural causes

The natural consequences of hunger, thirst and tiredness have their own natural remedies of eating, drinking and sleeping.

## *Treatment*

Treatments can take a variety of forms.

### MEDICINES

Medicines may be natural remedies from herbs, vegetables and minerals, but you may also be given homeopathic medicine or even conventional drugs.

### DIETARY REMEDIES

Diet is a very important part of Ayurvedic medicine. You will be advised to eat some foods and avoid others, depending on what you need to bring you back into balance and health. For example, you may be advised to eat meat and spices to raise your energy, or dairy products to lower your energy.

How you eat is also important. Ayurvedic medicine suggests that food should be eaten slowly and chewed well. Savouring and enjoying food is an important part of the process. In some situations, the practitioner may recommend fasting.

### PURIFICATION

The most common form of Ayuvedic purification therapy is known as 'Panchakarma', a five-fold therapy which includes:

- Saunas
- Laxatives/induced vomiting
- Enemas
- Nasal inhalations
- Blood letting.

### MASSAGE AND OILING

Special oils are used in Ayurvedic massage, and the massage itself is sometimes performed by two people at the same time, with each therapist taking one side of your body and working in harmony together.

Oiling may consist of a head or hand massage using specially selected oils – or it may be a gentle flow of oil onto the forehead. The flow of oil onto the forehead is particularly relaxing and can be helpful in serious complaints such as Alzheimer's or Parkinson's disease.

### COUNSELLING/TEACHING

The practitioner will also talk to you about the different things you can do to help bring yourself back into balance. This may take the form of changing your daily routine, doing special yoga exercises, meditating, or changing your diet. You may also be encouraged to change your attitudes towards life.

The Ayurvedic practitioner will probably draw up a treatment plan and discuss this with you.

## What is Ayurvedic medicine suitable for?

As Ayurveda is a complete system of medicine, it can be used for virtually any complaint. Looking specifically at conditions which are common in older people, Ayurvedic medicine has had particularly good results for people with arthritis and irritable bowel syndrome, as well as Parkinson's disease. It can also be helpful with back pain, prostate problems, depression, eye problems such as cataracts, bronchitis, myalgic encephalomyelitis (ME) and rheumatism.

### ADVANTAGES OF THIS FORM OF TREATMENT

- You will be given advice and guidance about your general lifestyle from what you eat, to how you exercise. Some of the treatments (such as oiling and massage) are very enjoyable.

### DISADVANTAGES OF THIS FORM OF TREATMENT

- You may be asked to change your lifestyle, your diet or exercise as part of the treatment.
- Some of the treatments (such as induced vomiting) are not at all enjoyable.

### SELF-TREATMENT

Ayurveda medicine is not suitable for treating yourself, you need to see an Ayurvedic practitioner. However, you may be asked to do some things to help yourself – such as learning meditation or yoga, changing your diet, taking regular exercise and so on.

## The Ayurvedic philosophy

Ayurveda is based on five elements:

- Earth
- Water
- Air
- Fire
- Ether (or space)

Every living cell contains these five elements

- The cell itself is mainly earth
- The liquid in the cell (cytoplasm) is water
- What happens in the cell is governed by fire
- The gases in the cell are mainly air
- The space the cell occupies represents ether

Since we are all made up of living cells, we have all five elements in our bodies, but some elements are more dominant than others. The Ayurvedic practitioner's task is to decide which of the elements are out of balance – and how to bring them back into balance.

The different constitutional types or doshas and their elements:

- **Pitta** – mainly fire, with water
- **Vata** – mainly ether, with air
- **Kapha** – mainly water, with earth

## Resources

*The Complete Illustrated Guide to Ayurveda.* Gopi Warrier and Deepika Gunawar, Element, 1997.

*The Book of Ayurveda.* Judith Morrison, Gaia Books, 1995.

*Ageless Body, Timeless Mind.* Deepak Chopra, Rider, 1993.

### THE AYURVEDIC HOSPITAL, LONDON

Only chronic, long-standing complaints can be treated at the Ayurvedic Hospital. There are no facilities for emergency treatments. Complaints treated include:

- Rheumatoid arthritis, gout and other auto-immune diseases
- Osteoarthritis, degenerative arthritis
- Hemiplegia, paraplegia
- General anxiety disorders/depression/obesity
- Diabetes
- Chronic pains, headache, migraine
- Parkinson's disease
- Alcoholism/addiction
- Coronary artery disease.

There are 30 beds. Patients are selected on the basis of the condition they suffer from and the ability of Ayurveda to cure it or at least give a better quality of life. People who are referred by their GP will be given a higher priority than people who apply by themselves. The hospital will insist on seeing your medical records and you must be under 75.

There are four Ayurvedic doctors and three Western doctors. The main treatments available at the hospital are herbal body massage, herbal steam bath, herbal oil dripping on head, herbal nasal drops, and enema with medicated oils. Yoga therapy is also available at the hospital. No charges are made for treatment, food, accommodation or medication.

A list of qualified practitioners is available from The Ayurvedic Company of Great Britain.

# Naturopathy

'Naturopathy' means being close to nature or benefiting from nature. It embraces several therapies which all support our natural ability to heal ourselves.

## *History of naturopathy*

The key idea behind naturopathy is that nature knows best, so its history dates right back to primitive times when we reacted instinctively to illness and disease. The first people to stop eating food to rest upset stomachs and sweat out fevers were all practising naturopathy. The therapy can trace its roots to the time of Hippocrates, around 400 BC, as it is based on Hippocratic principles (see box). It is also linked to Hygieia, the Goddess of health, who represented health through living in harmony with our own nature.

## Naturopathy's Hippocratic principles

- Only nature heals, providing it is given the opportunity to do so.
- Let food be your medicine and let medicine be your food.
- Disease is an expression of purification.
- All disease is one. (This means that all diseases are signals that we are out of balance.)

Modern naturopathy started in Germany by therapists such as Vincent Pressnitz (1799–1851) who believed in the miraculous healing power of water and developed what we now call hydrotherapy. Towards the end of the 19th century, a Bavarian monk Father Sebastian Kneipp (1824–1897) treated an American called Benedict Lust (1872–1945). Lust was so impressed with the water treatment he studied with Kneipp before returning to the US to form his own therapy which he called naturopathy.

Naturopathy became very popular in America and Germany in the 1920s. At its peak, America had 22 naturopathic colleges, but by the 1950s it was practically extinct. It started to revive in the 1960s and is now fully recognised in 18 states in America, where naturopathic doctors have the same status as conventionally trained doctors.

In Britain, naturopathy emerged in the beginning of the 20th century as 'the Nature Cure movement'. It became known as naturopathy towards the end of the 1920s. Naturopathy went into a decline in the 1950s and by 1961 the professional organisation merged with the osteopaths to become the British Naturopathic and Osteopathic Association. It almost sank without trace under the increasing popularity of osteopathy but, in 1992, the two organisations separated and the British Naturopathic Association was reborn.

Until recently, naturopathy has had a slightly old fashioned image, but this is in the process of changing and the naturopaths now have their own website. Naturopathic ideals have become increasingly accepted. For example, naturopaths have always focused on supporting health and preventing disease. This emphasis has become increasingly popular with governments, as reflected in their health awareness programmes such as stop smoking campaigns. In another sign of the increasingly naturopathic times, the lottery fund is currently spending £300 million on healthy living centres.

## What happens when you have a consultation?

During the first visit, you will be asked detailed questions about your current illness, past medical history, eating habits, lifestyle and stress levels. You may also be given a full physical examination which may include a chiropractic or osteopathic assessment to see if any of your joints are out of alignment.

Naturopaths use many different ways of finding out why you are ill and how you can get better. They may use iridology (seeing what is wrong with you by looking at the iris of the eye), allergy testing, applied kinesiology, and/or laboratory tests. The idea behind these tests is to find the root cause of your problems and the best way to treat them. You will probably be given some form of treatment and the naturopath will discuss a treatment plan that will be designed to help you to regain your health and vitality. If the practitioner needs the results of tests to draw up the treatment plan, then the plan can be discussed on your second visit.

## Treatment

Naturopaths use a number of different treatments.

### DIET AND FASTING

You may be asked to switch to a balanced, wholefood diet with a high percentage of raw vegetables and fresh fruit, or a special diet which will help your particular ailment. If you have allergies you may be advised to avoid certain foods such as dairy products and wheat.

The inner cleansing process of fasting allows the body to rest so that it can concentrate on healing itself from disease.

### STRUCTURAL ADJUSTMENT

The naturopath may use osteopathy, chiropractic, exercises and other techniques to balance and align your spine, muscles, ligaments and joints.

### HYDROTHERAPY

This covers a wide range of specific water treatments for particular health problems. For example, you may be advised to have hot and cold water footbaths for high blood pressure. The water treatments may include baths, packs, compresses, sprays, wet towels and douches.

### HEALTHY LIFESTYLE

Aspects of lifestyle include regular and appropriate exercise, cultivating a positive approach to life, and relaxation techniques. Naturopaths will also encourage you to avoid harmful substances such as nicotine and give you advice about looking after your body. This may include brushing your skin to remove dead skin and improve circulation.

### EDUCATION

The naturopath will explain the root cause of your disease to you and advise you about what you can do to help yourself.

## OTHER THERAPIES

You may also be given other forms of treatment which work in a naturopathic way, for example, dietary supplements, homeopathic remedies, Bach flower remedies, herbs or acupuncture.

## WHAT IS NATUROPATHY SUITABLE FOR?

Naturopathy heals the person, not the disease, so it is suitable for any complaint. Naturopaths are the equivalent of GPs in complementary medicine and they may refer you to other therapists – for example a homeopath or an osteopath – if you need specialist treatment.

Naturopathy can be particularly helpful if you want to improve your general level of health and vitality. It can be useful for chronic fatigue or ailments such as cancer where there has been a breakdown in the immune system. It can also be used to support the vital force during drug and surgery-based treatment.

Fasting is particularly effective at helping such problems as obesity, high blood pressure, arthritis and rheumatism, allergies and some psychiatric disorders.

## ADVANTAGES OF THIS FORM OF TREATMENT

- It is comprehensive. A naturopath will give you a thorough medical examination and attempt to get at the root cause of your symptoms.
- It helps you to learn about your own body and puts you in control of your health.

## DISADVANTAGES OF THIS FORM OF TREATMENT

- You may not want to change to a healthier lifestyle.

## SELF-TREATMENT

Many of the naturopathic principles such as eating a wholefood diet and having plenty of fresh air and exercise can be used without seeing a naturopath. However, if you are ill, or if you want a personal plan to improve your health, then it is best to consult a naturopath.

## What naturopaths expect from their treatment

Your health should improve, even though you may experience a 'healing crisis'. Such a crisis involves a return of old symptoms, usually in reverse order of their appearance. This is especially true of those symptoms which have been previously suppressed. Unpleasant as such an experience might be at the time, it is actually a signal that the body is dealing with the disease.

There is also likely to be a movement of the disease from the inside out – for example, asthma may clear up, but it is likely that eczema will return.

Homeopaths (and other natural therapists) have the same understanding of the healing process.

There are currently 310 naturopaths in the UK who are registered with the General Council and Register of Naturopathy. Training is four years full time.

# Herbal medicine

Herbal medicine is the use of plants or plant parts as medicine. It is also known as phytotherapy, phytomedicine or botanical medicine. The herbs in herbal medicine include leaves, stems, flowers, fruits, seeds, roots and bark.

## History of herbal medicine

The use of herbs as medicine is as old as humankind – perhaps even older when you consider that animals instinctively eat plants with healing properties. The earliest evidence of people using herbal remedies was found at a 60,000 year old Neanderthal burial site. Herbal medicine is mentioned in the Bible. 'The Lord hath created medicines out of the earth', we are told in Ecclesiastes chapter 28, while the psalmist sings, 'He causes herbs to grow for the service of man' (Psalm 104).

In ancient China, the mythical Shen Nong (divine father) would poison himself 80 times a day, but he was so skilled in herbal medicine that he always found the correct remedy. He recorded 365 'herbs' which included plant, animal and mineral substances.

The ancient Egyptians also used plant, animal and minerals for healing and had official schools of herbalists as early as 3000 BC. The slaves who built the pyramids chewed daily rations of raw garlic as a protection against infections. The Egyptians passed on their knowledge to the Greeks; Hippocrates himself was taught by Egyptian priest doctors.

Diascorides, a famous Greek doctor, travelled with the Roman armies in Asia and Europe where he learned a great deal about herbs and their uses. He recorded his findings in *De Materia Medica* in the first century AD, and it became one of the main medical textbooks for more than 13 centuries.

The Roman doctor Galen (130–201 AD) classified medicinal substances by a number of qualities including hot, cold, moist, dry or temperate (neutral). He matched these qualities in the plants to the qualities, characteristics and symptoms of the patient and prescribed accordingly. His methods became the basis for Western herbalism and his ideas are still being used today.

Herbalism as it is currently practised in Britain is partly the product of the oral tradition of wise women who collected and prescribed herbs and partly the result of the knowledge that was imported from the Roman Empire and North America.

The early settlers in North America in the 18th and 19th centuries relied heavily on herbal medicine as they were so far from civilisation. They had brought many of their own herbs, but also found familiar plants in the New World. There were many stories of trappers and other explorers falling ill and being treated by friendly native tribes. Ordinary settlers and the native Americans were quite neighbourly and used to trade with each other and swap ideas. Some of the early settlers specialised in using local herbs and native American lore for healing and set up their travelling medicine shows, and were known as the 'white Indian doctors'.

In pre-industrialised Britain, people went to the wise woman in the village who knew about the healing power of local herbs. During the industrial revolution, people moved into the rapidly expanding towns and started to rely on the new shops which were springing up offering medicines. Most minor complaints like headaches and stomach aches could be dealt with literally over the counter. But for something more serious, the counter flap would be lifted up and you would be taken to the back of the shop for treatment.

These herbal shops were so successful that they often had queues forming out into the street. They were particularly popular with working men who found that the treatments offered were cheaper and got them back to work more quickly than conventional doctors. Some of the treatments sound quite alarming and there are records of minor amputations and the use of emetics (medicine that is designed to make you vomit). Despite this, the shops were such a threat to the newly formed British Medical Association that herbalists were forced to form their own professional associations. Several regional associations were set up, joining forces in 1864 to become the National Association of Medical Herbalists. Jesse Boot of Nottingham, the man who started the Boots the Chemists empire, was one of the founder members.

Herbalists tended to be individualists who relied on a largely oral tradition. Forming an association meant that they had to find written ideas that they could all agree on. Books by Samuel Thomson and Albert Coffin provided perfect starting points. Thomson's original ideas were brought under the umbrella of the American Medical Association, and sank without trace. In England, however, those very same ideas survived because they became the founding philosophy of the National Association of Medical Herbalists. Right up to the late 1970s the training for herbalists in Britain was based on Thomson's principles and almost half the remedies taught were American. The National Association of Medical Herbalists is now called the National Institute of Medical Herbalists. Their debt to the past is acknowledged by their coat of arms with an Egyptian figure on one side and a native American in full head dress holding a bunch of herbs on the other.

# Two herbal heroes

**Samuel Thomson (1769–1843)** was brought up on a farm in New Hampshire and was introduced to herbs by Mrs Benton, who knew about American Indian herbs and healing. He was only a shepherd boy, but he learned how to read and write and wrote a book about what he had learned from Mrs Benton.

Thomson's message was simple: life and health are positive virtues that are to be protected or recovered through personal self sufficiency using the medicinal aids provided by God, whom he called the Maker. The book was a bestseller and Thomson became a popular figure, not only promoting his own views, but attacking those of the medical profession. He believed the medical approach, using blood letting, leeches and near fatal doses of poisonous ores such as arsenic, to be downright dangerous, and said so. The medical profession fought back. Thomson was dragged through the courts and accused of manslaughter and murder. He fought all the cases successfully – except one. On this last count, he was actually guilty of assault, having lost his temper and attacked one of his tormentors with a scythe.

While Thomson had his critics in the medical profession, he also inspired a huge following and his work inspired **eclecticism** and **physiomedicalism**. These were brought within the established American Medical Association and were swallowed up by scientific medicine.

We may never have heard of Thomson or physiomedicalism if it had not been for the fact that his ideas found their way to England and took root. This was thanks in part to **Albert Coffin** and his version of Thomson's book *Botanic Guide to Health*, published in 1847. Thomson's ideas were referred to as 'Thomsonian' in America, while Coffin's ideas about health became known by the strangely inappropriate title of 'Coffinism'.

## What happens when you have a consultation?

Seeing a herbalist will be quite similar to seeing your GP, except that you will see the herbalist for at least an hour for your first appointment. The herbalist will ask a lot of questions, and will want to know about:

- The problem you are immediately concerned with
- Any other health problems you are suffering from
- Your full medical history

The herbalist will also ask questions to enable them to build up a broad picture of your general health and lifestyle. These will include questions on the following topics:

- Your diet
- How much exercise you get
- The major stresses in your life
- Conditions which make you feel better
- Conditions which make you feel worse

The questions will be accompanied by a conventional physical examination. For example, if it is appropriate, the herbalist may take your blood pressure, and listen to your heart and chest. Some herbalists have had extra training in traditional Chinese medicine and may also use Chinese tongue and/or pulse diagnosis.

The herbalist will not only give you herbs, but may also make recommendations about changing your diet and lifestyle, or suggest relaxation techniques and exercises. You will be told how to take the herbs and how long it is likely to be before you feel better.

The herbs may come as tablets, pessaries, creams, ointments, compresses or even dried herbs which have to be boiled. You may be given a tincture with a mixture of four to ten herbs preserved in alcohol. Although some herbalists make their own tinctures, most will buy them from companies which satisfy stringent safety standards.

### ADVANTAGES OF HERBAL MEDICINE

- Because seeing a herbalist is similar to seeing a doctor, it is easy to accept and understand. You are being asked to do something that is very familiar: 'take this medicine, so many times a day'. In fact the whole rationale behind herbal treatment is easy to understand in conventional terms since it relies on the chemical constituents of the plants, just as ordinary doctors rely on the chemical ingredients in their medicine.

- You are also being given the herbalist's undivided attention for a considerable length of time – and this in itself can be quite a relief. A conventional doctor tries to understand what is 'wrong' and orders different tests to discover details of your disorder. But a herbalist is more concerned about you as an individual. The doctor will prescribe medicine for the disease, the herbalist will prescribe medicine for the person.

- The herbalist will be aiming to restore your body to balance in a very broad sense – looking at the sort of person you are in terms of your physical constitution, emotional type, and medical history.

- Herbal medicine tends to be gentle and will make you feel better in a fairly general way rather than just curing the specific symptoms that you are suffering from.

- The herbs are less likely to have damaging side-effects than conventional medicine. For example, dandelion leaf is a very effective diuretic (it helps you pass urine), similar to the drug frusemide. But while frusemide can cause problems because it lowers the body's potassium levels, dandelion leaves are naturally high in potassium. Aspirin is perhaps the best known example where the complete plant is safer than any single, active ingredient. Aspirin originally came from the salicylic acid in willow and meadowsweet (botanical name, *Filipendula ulmaria*). While aspirin is notorious for its potential side effect of damaging the stomach lining, meadowsweet is used to heal the same problem.

- Herbal medicine can often be used together with the medicine prescribed by your doctor.

- As you get better, your doctor may want to reduce your conventional medication.

## DISADVANTAGES OF THIS FORM OF TREATMENT

- Some forms of herbal medicine should not be used together with the medicine that is prescribed by your doctor. The effects could cancel each other out, or may even be dangerous. So it is important to see a properly qualified herbalist, and to tell the herbalist exactly what medicines you are taking from the doctor. It is also important to tell your doctor which herbs you are taking.

- The herbs themselves can taste quite awful.
- Just like conventional medicine, you have to remember to take the herbs. They won't work if you don't take them.
- You don't have to see the herbalist very often, which can be a disadvantage if you need ongoing emotional support.
- The herbs may not work quickly enough when the problem is life-threatening.

## What is herbal medicine suitable for?

The biggest study of herbal medicine so far has looked at its effect on osteoarthritis. This study was written up by Dr Wojciech Kielczynski and reported in *The European Journal of Herbal Medicine* in Autumn 1997. Hundreds of patients using herbal medicine had been monitored over several years, and the results showed a clear difference in terms of mobility and reduction in orthodox drugs taken.

Herbalism, like other forms of natural medicine, cannot reverse damage that has already been done, but it can help in the early stages of many diseases. This makes it important to see a herbalist when you first start to experience problems. For example:

- The early stages of heart failure with the first signs of breathlessness and water retention.
- A rise in blood pressure.
- Slight memory loss and a general slowing down of the mental faculties.

Because herbal medicine has a slow and general effect, it is not particularly suitable for life and death crises. Herbal medicine can be very effective in tackling flu and chest infections and the herbalist will use a variety of herbs to stimulate the immune system. But for more serious complaints such as pneumonia, more drastic measures are needed, and it is time to call in the GP.

Herbal medicine can be particularly good for complaints which have been going on for some time, where there is no irreversible physical damage. For example:

- Menopausal symptoms – skin dryness, brittle bones and hot flushes.
- Digestive problems – constipation, indigestion.
- Poor circulation – particularly where you have no specific symptoms except for feeling cold all the time.
- Leg ulcers – notoriously difficult to treat using orthodox medicine – can be very successfully treated with herbs, although they do need a lot of attention. The herbalist may prescribe a herbal ointment or a wash to use around the ulcer and may suggest exercise and hot and cold showers near the ulcer.
- Urinary tract infections such as cystitis – these respond well to herbal medicines with anti-inflammatory properties (but herbal medicine cannot help with mechanical problems such as weak sphincter muscles).

## How long does treatment take?

This varies enormously with the nature of the problem. You will normally be asked to visit the herbalist again, two weeks after your first appointment and then once a month for three to six months. You may be asked to carry on taking the medicine a bit longer and given suggestions of things you can do to help yourself.

The longer you have had the problem, the longer it will take to cure. With chronic problems like arthritis, it is likely to be three months or more before you start to notice a difference and you may have to wait six to nine months before seeing a big change. If your problem is an acute one, you may need to see the herbalist more frequently than for a long-standing condition. In acute situations such as flu or bronchitis, the process is much quicker, but still does not happen overnight. If bronchitis doesn't clear up within ten days, it's time to call in the GP.

### SELF-TREATMENT

Herbal medicine is perfect for self-treatment provided the problem isn't too serious or deep seated. If self-treatment does not work, consult a qualified medical herbalist.

If you are on any medication from your doctor, consult a medical herbalist rather than simply buying herbal remedies over the counter.

# Herbal hints

- If you have occasional sleeping problems drink a tea of lime flowers and hot water, half an hour before bed. It is also a good idea to have a warm bath with lavender oil.
- If you are going down with a chest infection, try garlic in honey. The daily dose is three teaspoons of honey with a clove of garlic in each teaspoon.
- If you are starting to develop arthritic pains in your joints, eat lots of parsley and drink nettle tea.
- For grazes and bruises try comfrey ointment for cuts and bruises – use calendula if there is redness and inflammation.
- For indigestion, try fennel tea, but crush up the seeds otherwise you will not get much benefit from the fennel.

# A bouquet of herbs

*Echinacea root (American coneflower root)*
This is a wonderful herb for stimulating the immune system and is good at preventing and treating bacterial and viral infections. But it should be used with caution. If you keep taking it as a preventative measure, you may be over-stimulating your immune system and so do more harm than good. Do not use it for longer than eight days at a time. If you need to keep taking echinacea, wait at least four days before repeating it.

If you are using it to treat an infection such as flu, you have to 'jump start' the immune system with hefty doses to have any effect. If you are seeing a herbalist anyway, it is cheaper to buy echinacea from them than to buy it at the healthfood shop.

*Garlic*
Garlic is more effective raw than cooked. If you are coming down with bronchitis you want the garlic to pass through your lungs, so you want the smelly breath that eating it gives you.

There has been considerable research which shows that garlic is also helpful in cardiovascular disease (high blood pressure, high levels of cholesterol etc). You want the garlic in your bloodstream, not your breath, so it is not necessary to have smelly breath and the garlic pearls you can buy in healthfood shops can be helpful.

*Ginger*
Although this is best known for calming morning sickness, it can also be a helpful stimulant for digestive problems and can be a good heart tonic.

*Ginkgo biloba*
Otherwise known as the maidenhair tree, this is the world's oldest living tree species and can be traced back more than 200 million years. It is often referred to as 'the living fossil'. In Germany and France extracts from Ginkgo biloba leaves are among the most commonly prescribed drugs and are available as tablets, liquid and as injections. It can be helpful for memory loss and a general lack of mental alertness. Herbalists may prescribe Ginkgo biloba for more serious problems such as signs of heart failure and the aftermath of strokes.

## Herb safety

Just because herbs are natural, does not automatically mean they are safe. After all, many plants such as the foxglove and deadly nightshade are poisonous if taken in large enough quantities. Almost anything can be dangerous if you take too much of it, so it is important to follow the directions given to you by your herbalist. Always tell your doctor if you are taking herbs – and tell your herbalist if you are taking medicines from the doctor. If you are taking medicine from the doctor, do not buy herbs from health food shop without checking with your doctor. The more serious the problem, the more important it is to see a qualified herbalist.

# Aromatherapy

Aromatherapy means what it says – it is the aroma from plants and trees which act as a therapy. You do not even have to be able to smell in order for the aroma to work its magic.

## *History of aromatherapy*

The word 'aromatherapy' was invented by the French chemist Rene Maurice Gattefosse who stumbled across this form of treatment when he plunged his badly burned hand into a container of lavender essence. His hand healed remarkably quickly without forming a blister or leaving a scar. He went on to treat wounded soldiers in World War I and discovered many other healing oils before writing his book, *Aromatherapie* (published in 1937).

French physician and biochemist Dr Jean Valnet and beautician Marguerite Maury took aromatherapy further. Valnet used essential oils to treat serious illnesses such as cancer, tuberculosis, and diabetes and Marguerite Maury developed techniques such as massage and various beauty and skin care treatments using essential oils. In fact modern aromatherapy came to Britain in the late 1950s through beauticians rather than through medical channels.

Although Gattefosse, Maury and Valnet were the 20th century pioneers of aromatherapy, people have been using the healing power of smell since ancient times when healing was a matter for the spirit as well as the body. For example, Ayurvedic medicine includes one of the oldest known books on plants which not only mentions aromatic materials such as sandalwood, ginger, myrrh, cinnamon and coriander, but also indexes their various uses for both religious and medicinal purposes. Native Americans traditionally burn sage and sweetgrass to cleanse and purify, Buddhists burn incense and Roman Catholic priests burn frankincense.

In ancient Egypt, each of the gods was allotted a particular fragrance with which their statues were sometimes anointed. The pharaohs themselves were anointed with specially prepared aromatic ointments for times of prayer, war and love. The Egyptians also used aromatic substances in the embalming process for both humans and animals.

## Perfume

The world 'perfume' comes from the Latin *per fumum* meaning 'through the smoke', and refers to the burning of incense.

The Bible cites many references to incense together with the use of plant oils and ointments.

A Greek, Megallus formulated a perfume called megaleion which was well known throughout Greece. It not only smelled good, it also helped heal wounds and reduce inflammation.

The use of essential oils spread from Egypt throughout the Middle East, ancient Greece and Rome. Essential oils and flower waters came to Britain via the Romans and later from soldiers returning home from the Crusades. Essential oils were used in mainstream medicine throughout the 16th and 17th centuries.

## Healing qualities of plants

In 1576, the Swiss alchemist Paracelsus wrote *The Great Surgery Book* in which he suggested that the main role of alchemy was to develop medicines, especially *quinta essenta* (the healing extracts from plants) claiming that the essential oils were the most highly desirable part of a plant.

Many people believed that the wearing of plants disinfected the air, giving them protection against infection. The plague claimed so many victims that it is tempting to dismiss this belief as mere superstition but, as the box below shows, some essential oils do in fact have antiseptic properties.

## Antiseptic aromatherapy

Professor Griffon, a member of the French academy of pharmacy, made up a blend of seven essential oils (cinnamon, clove, lavender, peppermint, pine, rosemary and thyme) in an aerosol spray and studied their antiseptic effect on the surrounding air. He found that bacteria and moulds were destroyed within 30 minutes. (*The Practice of Aromatherapy*, by Jean Valnet, Daniel, 1980)

In the late 18th century, people turned to man-made perfumes. The use of essential oils and herbs declined, only to be reborn when Gattefosse, Maury and Valnet developed aromatherapy in France. Aromatherapy was brought to Britain through beauticians such as Shirley Price (whose book *Aromatherapy for Practitioners* was published by Churchill Livingstone in 1995). But it is increasingly becoming accepted as a therapy rather than just a pleasant experience. Indeed, according to Shirley Price, nurses and other healthcare workers have been so impressed with the benefits of aromatherapy that it rapidly became the most widely used complementary therapy in the National Health Service, being well received in hospitals, residential homes, and hospices.

## Distilling essential oils

The Roman doctor Dioscorides may have invented the distillation method of producing essential oils. He had cooked some pears between two plates in the oven. When they cooled, the inquisitive doctor tasted the liquid which had formed under the top plate. To his surprise it both smelled and tasted of pears, and he experimented with other fruits and plants to produce more of this delicious 'spirit' as he called it.

## What happens when you have a treatment?

The first step is a consultation. Apart from wanting to know about your current symptoms, the aromatherapist will take a full medical history. He or she will want to know what medicines you are taking and will ask you a series of questions to get an idea about your general lifestyle, including:

- Your diet
- Your emotional state
- The factors which cause you stress
- How much exercise you take.

Based on this consultation, the aromatherapist will then choose up to five different oils.

If your problems are stress-related, the treatment may consist of a full body aromatherapy massage. This can be a wonderfully relaxing experience, and you may find yourself eager for more. Many people who have an aromatherapy massage late in life wonder why on earth they had not tried it sooner.

If you do not like the idea of having a full body massage, the aromatherapist may suggest that you just have your hands and feet done, or your head, neck and shoulders.

Aromatherapists may also tell you what you can do to help yourself and may suggest you use the oils in a bath or as a lotion. They may also give you advice on preventative measures and health care to help you improve your general well-being.

Although many people in Britain think of aromatherapy massage when they think of aromatherapy, there are many other ways of using the essential oils – for example in lotions, ointments, compresses, gargles and inhalations. The oils can also be used as medicines in a form of the therapy known as 'aromatology' (the medical version of aromatherapy) which doesn't include massage and is mainly practised in France.

## What is aromatherapy suitable for?

Aromatherapy is helpful for circulatory, emotional, muscular and psychological problems, particularly insomnia and restlessness. It can also help you reduce your need for medication – particularly for painkillers, sleeping tablets, tranquillisers and anti-depressants. It can also help you cope with pain.

After a series of aromatherapy treatments you may need less medication. There are two reasons for this:

- You may be feeling better, and so need less medicine.
- Aromatherapy can affect your medicine by making it more powerful. This is known as a *potentising effect*.

It can also interfere with medication so always check with your GP before having aromatherapy. It is also important to discuss the dose of any prescribed medicines with your doctor – do not change the dose yourself without medical advice.

Healthcare professionals are increasingly recognising the value of aromatherapy oils in situations where pharmaceutical medicines have little to offer. For example, where drugs have caused side-effects, aromatherapy can be helpful in easing these without the need to resort to still more medicines.

Aromatherapy oils can be helpful in alleviating symptoms of people with Alzheimer's disease, especially where there is frequent or constant movement, wandering and searching behaviour. It can also calm and relieve anxiety and rosemary can improve memory. Shirley Price (see the Resources section on page 87) gives some interesting case studies for the use of essential oils. Aromatherapy has also been found to be helpful in hospice situations where the essential oils can have an uplifting and calming effect on patients and their loved ones, as well as on healthcare professionals themselves.

Conditions and situations in which aromatherapy can be particularly helpful include:

- Alzheimer's disease
- Parkinson's disease
- Rheumatoid arthritis

- Cancer care
- Terminal illness
- Bereavement
- Before and after surgery
- Intensive care
- Burns
- Mental health care.

### ADVANTAGES OF THIS FORM OF TREATMENT

- Aromatherapy massage is enjoyable, the relaxing power of touch is very soothing to the nervous system. Touching and being touched fulfils a very basic human need.
- Aromatherapy is a non-invasive therapy which is easy to administer and can be almost as pleasant to give as to receive.
- Compared to orthodox medicines, aromatherapy oils are very cheap because there are no research costs added to the cost of production.

### DISADVANTAGES OF THIS FORM OF TREATMENT

- Aromatherapy doesn't suit everybody.
- Aromatherapy massage has the same disadvantages of a conventional massage. Not everyone likes the idea of massage, not everyone likes to be stroked or touched.
- It is not a good idea to use aromatherapy oils if you have some illnesses or are taking certain types of drugs. For example, there are some oils which can bring on epilepsy if you have a history of epilepsy. This is one of the reasons why it is best to see a qualified aromatherapist, rather than do it yourself.

### SELF-TREATMENT

One of the reasons for the increasing popularity of aromatherapy is that it is so easy to use. However, there are potential difficulties in the do-it-yourself approach:

- The little bottles the oils come in can be difficult to open.
- It can be hard to see the drops and count them for the right dose.
- Choosing the right oils or the right combination of oils can also be tricky.

It is important to buy the best quality essential oils. The cheap oils may smell fine, but are not suitable if you want to use them therapeutically.

It is easy to confuse the essential oil (which you shouldn't take internally) with food products which are perfectly safe. For example, peppermint essential oil shouldn't be eaten, but oil of peppermint can be. It is also easy to confuse essential oils with perfumes or perfume water, for example, natural essential lavender oil is quite different from lavender fragrances which can be made from synthetic materials.

Some essentials oils can be dangerous if you have too much of them, particularly if you have a tendency towards high blood pressure, or have problems with your nervous system. Some oils can burn or irritate the skin if used in the bath – clove and lemongrass oil are both examples of this. The easiest way of using the oils yourself is to consult an aromatherapist and ask them to make up a mixture for you in an easy to open container. Then you can do-it-yourself – provided that you always follow two golden rules:

- **Rule One: Don't use too much**
  Don't be tempted to say the more the merrier because the oils can have the opposite effect if used in too high a dose. For example, lavender can be relaxing and cure headaches and nausea at the correct dose, but can actually cause agitation, headaches and nausea if you use too much. The very young and the very old should only use **half** the normal recommended dose of any oil. You should also only use half doses if you are ill, no matter what your age.

- **Rule Two: Don't apply directly to the skin**
  The oils should be used in a carrier oil or diluted in water. If the skin is broken or ulcerated, they should be applied in a cream or lotion around the wound, not directly on it. Hospitals use essential oils in water sprays on wounds.

## WHICH OILS TO USE

There are many oils to choose from. Here are a few which are particularly suitable and safe for home use.

## Lavender

Lavender is one of the most useful of all the aromatherapy oils. It is best known for its calming, relaxing qualities. It is particularly useful for burns and insect bites and should be in everyone's first aid kit. It is also useful as an antiseptic and for pain relief, particularly if the pain is made worse because of stress.

## Chamomile

Another calming, relaxing oil, chamomile makes a good combination with lavender. It is excellent for insomnia. Chamomile is also a good anti-inflammatory for muscular and rheumatic aches and pains.

## Lemon

This is particularly helpful if you have painful, arthritic joints because it detoxifies and has an uplifting effect. It also acts as a natural antibiotic, so it is helpful if you have a cold. Mix with chamomile for the best effect.

## Sandalwood

Sandalwood is effective for relaxation and treating insomnia. It can also be used for dry skin and to help heal wounds.

## Ginger

Useful for improving the circulation, nausea and digestive problems, ginger has a warming effect. It can be used as an inhalation or put in a foot bath.

## Rose otto

Rose otto has a calming effect for insomnia, stress and skin problems. It can be used in a bath, with a diffuser or in cream for skin problems.

### ADMINISTERING THE OILS

Two or even three oils used in combination are more powerful than using just one on its own.

## Baths

There is something luxurious about stepping into an aromatherapy bath and breathing in the scented vapours, knowing that it will be doing you good. Use four drops of oil in a bath full of water. You can mix the oils with a little bit of single cream or powdered milk and water so that the oil does not just float on top.

## Footbaths

Sitting quietly with your feet in aromatherapy water is surprisingly soothing and relaxing. Just use three drops of essential oil to a bowl of water. In the summer use cool, tepid water to reduce swelling, in the winter use warm water to improve circulation.

## Inhalations

This is not suitable for people who suffer from asthma because they may choke on the steam.

A bowl of hot water with essential oils can be helpful in easing cold symptoms. Use 1–2 drops of lavender and 1–2 drops of lemon essential oil in a bowl of very hot water and breathe in the vapours.

It is also a good idea to use oils in a bowl of hot water and let the aroma diffuse into the room. This is particularly helpful for stress, insomnia, anxiety, fear, and emotional problems.

Another way of inhaling is to put essential oil on your pillow. Put a drop or two onto a cotton ball or scrunched up tissue and tape it to the pillow – it is wonderful for insomnia. If you do not like it or it is too much for you, then it is easy to pull it off and throw it away without making the whole pillow smell.

## Lotions and creams for pain relief

Lavender, chamomile, ginger, eucalpytus, black pepper and rosemary can all be used in lotions and creams for pain relief (see the box). Do not use rosemary if you suffer from heart problems or epilepsy.

## Residential care homes and hospices

Although aromatherapy can be used in residential care homes and hospices, it needs to be used with some sensitivity. If the oils are used as a vaporiser in a room, it can affect the mood or health of all the people in the room – not always for the better. For example, when red thyme is inhaled it can cause aggression. However, most essential oils are perfectly safe and may be more pleasant than other smells.

---

# Recipes and suggestions

*Foot balms*
These can be helpful if you suffer from cold feet and bad circulation. Use an ordinary, unperfumed base cream, such as E45 and add lavender and ginger and/or black pepper. One drop of oil to one teaspoon of cream or eight drops of oil to a 50ml pot.

*Dry skin*
Choose from rose otto, geranium, chamomile, lavender, and frankincense in an unperfumed base cream. Use a total of eight drops to 50mls of base cream, or one drop per teaspoon. For a luxurious beauty cream try four drops of rose otto and four drops of frankincense in 50mls of unperfumed base cream. You can also use calendula cream as a base.

*Stress related headaches*
Try leaving a bowl of hot water with a few drops of lavender oil to scent the room. You can also can apply the lavender oil to your temples and forehead. Use one drop of lavender to one teaspoon (5ml) of almond oil and dab it on your temples. Alternatively use a face flannel as a cold compress by soaking the flannel in two drops of lavender in tepid water and holding it across your forehead.

*Arthritic pain*
Use lavender, chamomile and lemon essential oils mixed into an unperfumed base cream or lotion. Use eight drops of essential oil to 50 mls of cream or lotion. Creams and lotions get easily absorbed into the skin, so you don't have to massage vigorously.

## Resources

*Aromatherapy An A–Z*, by Patricia Davis. Daniel, 1995 (revised edition).

*The Practice of Aromatherapy*, by Dr Jean Valnet. Daniel, 1980.

*Aromatherapy for Health Professionals*, by Shirley Price and Len Price. Churchill Livingstone, 1995.

'Aromatherapy for Elder Care', by Laraine Kyle. *International Journal of Aromatherapy* 1998/99 vol 9 no 4.

# 5

# Physical Therapies

## Introduction

Imagine the body as a car. The better you look after it with regular servicing, the better it will work and the longer it will run. The physical therapies are concerned with servicing our physical structure, looking after our muscles, bones and joints and keeping them in good working order, minimising wear and tear.

The physical therapies focus on our physical frame, the part of our body that enables us to stand upright and move – our bones, muscles and ligaments. They also include our skin, the part of our body which keeps us together and separates us from the rest of the world.

Although this chapter is about the therapies that touch us physically, they also affect us energetically, emotionally and have an impact on our internal organs.

If someone or something hits you, or if you have a sudden shock, your body reacts automatically. Your muscles will clench, and you will turn away from the danger. The longer you live, the more often your body will have to react to the various assaults that life throws at you. Some of the traumas are real, some are just imagined as your body remembers what has happened in the past – and fears what may happen in the future. For example, I had a car crash while driving along a country lane over 30 years ago, and my body still tenses up when I see an approaching car if I am driving in the country.

Our bodies remember our accidents and try to protect us from getting into the same situation again. Unfortunately, this isn't very helpful as tensing muscles and contracting and turning away from imagined dangers just makes us tense and twisted. The physical therapies help us by releasing the pain and tension from the past as well as the present.

The physical therapies also help us to move freely – and movement is important because it helps us to keep active. The more active you are – the more you walk and exercise, the less stiff you feel, and you will sleep better and feel better. Of course the better you feel, the more you will be able to move, and the more active you feel, the more exercise you will be able to take. It is a virtuous circle that can easily turn into a vicious one if you do not feel able to move without pain. The physical therapies help you to keep moving with minimum wear and tear and discomfort.

Sometimes it can feel as if your body has become tightly wound up with the stress of everyday living – if this is the case, then let one of the physical therapies unwind that tightness. The physical therapies also tend to be relaxing – the perfect antidote to stress.

The physical therapies are all concerned with touch – and although they may mainly be concerned with our physical health and well-being they all 'touch us' at an emotional level as well. In the case of massage and zero balancing this is a very important part of the healing process.

Touch can also be an important way of nurturing ourselves as we get older, particularly if we are seldom touched by loved ones, if we are suffering from some discomfort or have to undergo medical procedures where touch becomes associated with discomfort.

The therapies covered in this section include:

- **Manipulative therapies,** with contact focused on the bones and joints (osteopathy; chiropractic).
- **'Soft tissue' therapies,** where touch is focused on our skin and muscles (massage; biodynamic massage).
- Therapies where the physical touch affects other parts of the body through **energy channels**, otherwise known as **meridians** (acupressure; shiatsu; reflexology).
- **Kinesiology,** in which contact is focused on the muscles (but it is also concerned with all the ways in which we can become stronger or weaker).

- **Zero balancing,** in which the first contact is focused on the bones and joints (but it can also have a profound affect on our energy and emotions).

In less than a decade, the physical therapies have been increasingly welcomed into the National Health Service. In 1994, the Clinical Standards Advisory Group's Committee on Back Pain recommended that there should be earlier access to the manipulative therapies. In 1996, the Royal College of General Practitioners issued guidelines for GPs, recommending manipulative treatment within the first six weeks for patients with low back pain.

# Osteopathy

The word osteopathy comes from the Greek words *osteon* (bone) and *pathos* (to suffer), so it literally means 'suffering of the bone'.

Osteopaths diagnose and treat mechanical problems in the body's framework of bones, joints, muscles and ligaments. Osteopaths use a range of techniques including massage, joint mobilisation and manipulation. They also provide advice on posture and lifestyle.

## History of osteopathy

An American doctor, Andrew Taylor Still (1828–1917) developed osteopathy in the mid-1870s and turned the bone setter's art into a science. He was an army doctor in the American civil war, but he felt powerless to help soldiers with wounds which got infected after battles and operations. The medicine of the day was equally ill-equipped at dealing with the epidemics which killed so many people after the war, including his own young wife and three of his children who died during an epidemic of spinal meningitis.

Still was deeply disillusioned with the medicine of the time and he thought carefully about the whole process of disease and health. He had studied engineering as well as human anatomy, so perhaps it is not surprising that he thought of the body as a machine, a mechanism that could be manipulated to restore balance and cure illness. Still believed that when the structure of the body was sound, it would work just like a well-tuned engine, with the minimum of wear and tear. He came to the conclusion that many illnesses are caused by a part of the body's structure coming out of alignment and that the doctor's role was to trace and treat the mechanical imbalance that lies behind the disease process.

At first, there was strong opposition to Still's ideas, but now osteopathy is an accepted part of modern medicine, particularly in the US where there are 15 specialised osteopathic medical schools.

Dr Martin Littlejohn studied with Still and set up the British School of Osteopathy in London in 1917. There are now five osteopathic schools in Britain and it has become one of the most accepted forms of complementary medicine.

## What happens when you have a consultation?

The osteopath will ask about your current complaint, as well as past problems relating to your health including accidents and surgery. You may also be asked other questions which will give the osteopath a broader picture of what is happening in your life and help them understand the most likely cause of your problems.

Osteopaths will also ask about other treatments you may be having and give you a physical examination. This will include asking you to move. For example, you may be asked to walk for a few steps or bend to one side and then the other. Having assessed the problem, the osteopath will then work out a course of action which may include asking for an x-ray, referring you to another practitioner or osteopathic treatment itself.

The osteopath will ask you to relax and may massage the area that needs treatment before applying a swift but gentle thrust to a joint to restore normal movement. If you have osteoporosis or are frail, osteopaths may use other techniques instead, such as passive movements where they move different joints in your body for you. You may also be given exercises and advice to follow at home.

The first treatment will probably take an hour, with follow-up treatments taking 30 minutes to an hour.

Your problems, particularly back problems, may feel easier immediately after treatment, but sometimes there may be a healing reaction. There may be a soreness where the osteopath has been working, or there may be a temporary worsening of your symptoms. This is a normal part of the healing process, but if you are concerned, you should contact your osteopath.

You may only need a few treatments, but some people benefit from weekly sessions for a while, followed by an occasional session every few months.

## What is osteopathy suitable for?

Low back pain and neck pain account for more than half of an osteopath's workload.

### ACCIDENTS AND FALLS

Osteopathy is particularly helpful where problems start after an accident – even if the accident happened many years ago. You may have forgotten the original accident, but the trained hands of an osteopath can often feel the effects on the body, years after the event, and osteopathic treatment can release the tension and strains from the past. This not only helps with pain, but it can also give you more energy as your body no longer has to cope with the stress of compensating after the original trauma.

### OPERATIONS

Osteopathy can speed recovery after surgery – particularly after hip replacements.

### HEADACHES

Osteopathy can be particularly effective in relieving the kind of tension headaches which are caused by contraction of the small muscles at the base of the skull.

## ARTHRITIS

Osteopathy can bring some relief from the early symptoms of osteoarthritis 'wear and tear'. As you get older, the joints that have been damaged by accidents and falls may become arthritic, and are most likely to be helped by osteopathic treatment.

## INTERNAL SYMPTOMS

Because of the effect that aligning the bones can have on other parts of the body, osteopathy may also be helpful for internal problems such as digestive problems, breathing problems and heart disease. Osteopathy can help in a more general ways such as improving circulation in the legs and giving you more mobility.

## ADVANTAGES OF THIS FORM OF TREATMENT

- Osteopaths have a very deep understanding of the mechanics of our backs and the skeletal system as a whole. It is the ideal way of treating mechanical problems such as a backache, particularly when this has been caused by an accident.
- Because osteopathy can help you to stay mobile, it can help you to help yourself stay fit by enabling you to carry on walking and doing the things that you enjoy.

## DISADVANTAGES OF THIS FORM OF TREATMENT

- Some people find that once the skeleton is back in alignment, it can easily slip out of alignment again. Sometimes the more treatments you have, the more easily this may happen if the ligaments get looser.
- Osteopathy can't turn the clock back completely. If you have arthritis, for example, osteopathic treatment may improve circulation around the joint, improve mobility and slow the rate of deterioration in the joint, but it cannot give you a new joint.

## SELF-TREATMENT

Osteopathy is not suitable for self-treatment or first aid, although the osteopath may suggest exercises for you to do at home.

It takes between four and five years full time study to become an osteopath. There are currently 2000 registered osteopaths in the UK, and another 800 who are going through the registration process.

# Cranial osteopathy

Cranial osteopathy is a very gentle and subtle form of osteopathic treatment

## History of cranial osteopathy

Cranial osteopathy was invented by William Garner Sutherland (1873–1954) who had learned ordinary osteopathy from its creator, Andrew Taylor Still. Sutherland was fascinated by the skull, particularly the cranial bones which come together in joints known as sutures. He had learned from Still that every structure had a function, and every function had a structure, what then was the purpose of these very fine joints that seem to be fused together?

He discovered that the bones in the skull actually did move very slightly – and so does the bone at the base of the spine, which is known as the sacrum. By experimenting on himself he found that these tiny movements allow what he called the primary respiratory mechanism. This is the gentle ebb and flow of the body's fluids and tissues – particularly the cerebrospinal fluid. He found that when the normal rhythm of these fluids are disrupted, then it can cause all sorts of problems from headaches to tinnitus. Cranial osteopaths use the gentlest possible touch to release the joints and help the fluids to return to their normal, natural rhythm.

Cranial osteopathy has become increasingly popular in Britain in recent years as both osteopaths and their clients appreciate this gentle way of working.

## What happens when you have a treatment?

Cranial osteopathy is practised by osteopaths, and so most of the session will be the same as an ordinary osteopathic session. When the therapist uses cranial osteopathy, you may feel sensations of pressure or warmth under their hands or elsewhere. It can feel as if the tension is being drawn out of your body and is deeply relaxing.

## What is cranial osteopathy suitable for?

Cranial osteopathy may be used for any of the complaints that ordinary osteopathy is used for, but it is particularly useful for head injuries and headaches, tinnitus (ringing in the ears) colitis, urinary incontinence, Bell's palsy, carpel tunnel syndrome and sciatica.

### ADVANTAGES OF THIS FORM OF TREATMENT

- It is very gentle and relaxing.
- You may find that it helps with your general energy levels and sleep patterns.

### DISADVANTAGES OF THIS FORM OF TREATMENT

- There may be some brief emotional or physical discomfort as old traumas rise to the surface for healing.

### SELF-TREATMENT

This therapy is not suitable for treating yourself.

# Chiropractic

The name of this therapy comes from the Greek words, *kheir* meaning hand and *praktikos* meaning practical. Chiropractic is a method of adjusting the bones in your body in order to relieve pain and restore movement. Chiropractors believe that keeping your spine in alignment will help your body's nerve supply to work efficiently.

## History of chiropractic

A caretaker called Harvey Lillard had been working in a cramped, stooping position when he felt a click in his back and became deaf. In 1865, some 17 years later, American healer Daniel David Palmer adjusted some of the small bones in Harvey Lillard's spine which cured both his backache and his deafness.

Palmer's theory behind this dramatic recovery was that when a part of the skeleton presses against the nerves, it can create problems in other parts of the body. A year after his first chiropractic adjustment, Palmer was arrested for practising medicine without a medical licence. Despite huge opposition from the medical establishment, he opened the first School of Chiropractic 33 years later and strangely enough five of the first fifteen graduates were also medical doctors.

The conflict between chiropractic and the medical establishment was finally resolved when a US judge decided that chiropractic was not medicine, but a discipline in its own right. Palmer's son, BJ Palmer refined his father's techniques and introduced the use of x-rays for more accurate diagnosis of spinal misalignments. Today, chiropractic is the third largest independent primary healing profession in the Western world after medicine and dentistry.

## Chiropractic in Britain

| | |
|---|---|
| 1925 | British Chiropractic Association formed |
| 1965 | Anglo European College of Chiropractic opened in Bournemouth (the first chiropractic college outside America) |
| 1972 | The McTimoney Chiropractic School was founded by John McTimoney |
| 1988 | Anglo European College of Chiropractic became the first complementary medicine college to offer a validated degree course in the UK |

## McTimoney chiropractic

John McTimoney established his practice in Oxfordshire in 1951 and developed a new approach to chiropractic which is now taught at the McTimoney Chiropractic College.

McTimoney uses a slightly different technique to adjust the bones: one hand is placed over the bone to be adjusted and given a glancing strike with the other hand. This gives energy to the bone and tissues which the body can use to re-set its skeletal structure. You may hear the noise of the two hands smacking together, but you are unlikely to be aware of the manipulation itself.

McTimoney chiropractors say that this technique does not stretch the ligaments surrounding the bones, thus minimising the risk of the spine coming out of alignment again.

In practice, there are fewer differences between McTimoney and ordinary chiropractors than you may think as they use each other's techniques.

## What happens when you have a consultation?

You will be asked about your current problems and details of your medical history, paying particular attention to any accidents and surgery you may have had. The chiropractor will then look at your posture and examine you, feeling for areas of muscle spasm, pain and tenderness, and find out which joints are moving properly and which are not. Some chiropractors also take x-rays, or ask for x-rays to be taken at your local hospital. All chiropractors are fully trained in the use of x-rays to help them decide which joints need adjusting.

The chiropractor will then decide on a course of treatment and you may have to come back for another visit for the treatment itself. The treatment is known as a chiropractic adjustment or manipulation.

You will be asked to strip down to your underwear, and offered a loose, comfortable robe to wear. You may have to stand, sit or lie on a couch for the treatment. When the chiropractor works on your body, you may be moved into different positions. For example, if you have a painful back, you may be asked to lie on your side, and the chiropractor may turn the upper spine one way and the lower spine the other way, exposing the vertebra that needs adjusting. The chiropractor feels the vertebra and using a little pressure, takes the joint to the end of its normal range of movement. Then the joint is given a sharp tap, directing a physical force into the spine, which allows it to spring back into position. The force used should not be painful, but it is often accompanied by a loud click.

The click or popping noise is what happens when a bubble of gas pops as the two surfaces of a joint are moved apart quickly and there is a sudden change of pressure within the joint space. The chiropractor will re-examine you and the joint should now be moving more freely, and because the muscles have been relaxed, the whole area should be more flexible. Some people feel better immediately, others may experience aching, soreness and stiffness later that day or the day after as the body adjusts.

## The difference between chiropractic and osteopathy

The most obvious difference between chiropractors and osteopaths is that chiropractors are trained to use x-rays.

The manipulations that chiropractors and osteopaths do are also different. Chiropractors tend to work directly with the bones, osteopaths also work with the soft tissues (muscles, tendons, ligaments etc).

Chiropractors expect benefits to flow from proper alignment improving the way the nerves work.

Osteopaths expect benefits from improving the circulation of the blood.

The first consultation takes about half an hour, but the treatment itself can be as quick as five minutes or as long as an hour, depending on your condition. The chiropractor may suggest exercises that will also help.

You may need five or six visits over a two to three week period. Generally, the longer you have had the problem, the more treatments you may need to put it right, although you should experience some improvement quite quickly. Chiropractors often suggest you come back every few months for check ups and to keep your joints moving freely.

## What is chiropractic suitable for?

Chiropractic treatment can relieve pain and discomfort and increase mobility. Its aims are to improve function, alignment, and mobility of the joints.

### What chiropractic can improve

- Function – the way a part of the body works
- Alignment – making sure everything is in the right place
- Mobility – ease of movement, flexibility

In the process, chiropractic releases the stress and strain on the body's nervous system and relieves pain. All of this can be particularly useful for several complaints which are common in older people.

Chiropractic is particularly suitable for:

- Neck pain
- Back pain
- Chest or abdominal pain
- Shoulder, arm, wrist and hand pain
- Leg, knee, ankle and foot pain
- Headache or migraine
- Poor circulation
- After-effects of operations, accidents, falls and bumps
- General symptoms of declining health, including poor mobility.

By keeping the body aligned, treatment can help to reduce further damage.

### ADVANTAGES OF THIS FORM OF TREATMENT

- It is one of the most accepted and widely used forms of natural medicine.
- Chiropractors are specialists and have a profound understanding of the bone structure and the way in which it affects the nerves and joint pain.

- It is satisfying to hear the joints 'pop' – you really feel that something has happened.

#### DISADVANTAGES OF THIS FORM OF TREATMENT

- The more chiropractic adjustments you have, the more you may need as your ligaments may loosen and the more likely it is that the bones may slip out of alignment again.
- Some people do not like the popping noise.

#### SELF-TREATMENT

Chiropractic is not suitable for self-treatment, although you may be asked to do exercises to help your recovery and prevent problems recurring.

# Massage

The word massage comes from the Arabic *masah* which means to stroke with the hand. Massage is the manipulation of the soft tissues of the body using a variety of movements and sequences. It is a formal form of touch – touch with intent.

## History of massage

Apes groom each other, animals lick their wounds and humans rub aching joints or muscles – these are all instinctive forms of massage. The earliest written record of massage appears in a Chinese book dating from about 2700 BC. Ancient Egyptian papyri also record the use of massage and the Greeks and Romans used massage as a curative and preventative therapy as well as for pleasure.

For centuries, massage has been an important part of the main systems of traditional medicine such as Ayurvedic medicine, traditional Chinese medicine and naturopathic medicine. In Europe, the most popular form of massage is Swedish massage. It is called Swedish massage because of the work of the fencing master Per Henrik Ling (1776–1839). Ling developed a system of massage which classified the massage strokes in terms of pressure, friction, vibration, percussion and rotation. Ling's work resulted in an institute being set up in

Stockholm and in 1838 a Swedish institute was opened in London, followed by other institutes in Russia, France and America.

There was a big upsurge of interest in massage during the 1960s as its beneficial effects on the emotions became more widely recognised. In the 1970s it became even more popular as people increasingly saw massage as a way of dealing with stress and many new forms were invented.

According to *The Encyclopaedia of Complementary Medicine*, there are over 100 different methods that can be classified under massage therapy, and about three quarters of them are less than 20 years old (see box) Although there are many new forms of massage, Swedish massage is still the most common.

## Some different types of massage therapies

- Swedish massage
- Deep tissue massage
- Manual lymph drainage
- Biodynamic massage
- Aromatherapy massage
- Shiatsu

Nurses learned massage in the first part of the 20th century and physiotherapists still learn massage as part of their training. Unfortunately, physiotherapists rarely have much time to use this skill in the normal part of practice within the NHS. But in the past few years, there has been increasing interest in the therapeutic use of massage and many nurses have trained as massage therapists and non-medically qualified massage therapists have started to work in NHS surgeries (see Section Three of this book).

## What happens when you have a treatment?

> When receiving a good massage, a person usually falls into a mental-physical state that is difficult to describe. It is like entering a special room until now locked and hidden away; a room the very existence of which is likely to be familiar only to those who practise some kind of meditation.
>
> George Downing, *The Massage Book*.

The therapist will ask you a few questions about your medical history and about any particular problems the massage should focus on – and what to avoid. You may want the person treating you to avoid areas that are sensitive to touch such as any infections, inflammations or current injuries. You also need to mention varicose veins, which the therapist may avoid totally or touch very lightly. If you have cancer, the therapist may avoid the affected area altogether.

The massage therapist will ask you to take off as many clothes as you feel comfortable with. If you don't feel comfortable about taking your clothes off, say so, and the therapist can concentrate on your hands and feet and perhaps your neck and shoulders. If you prefer not to remove your clothes, you may be happier with a form of massage that can be done fully clothed (such as shiatsu) or some other form of physical therapy such as zero balancing.

The therapist will normally leave the room while you undress unless you specifically ask for help. You will lie down on a comfortable massage couch, and your body will be covered over with towels. While working on different parts of your body, the therapist will uncover only the part which is being treated.

If it is difficult for you to get on the couch or lie flat, tell your therapist who will help to make you comfortable. For example, you may need plenty of cushions, help getting onto the couch or you may prefer to stay in a chair.

The massage itself may consist of a number of different strokes, depending on your own particular needs and the style of massage your therapist uses. The strokes may be:

- Close to the surface, with flowing or gliding strokes in the direction of the heart.
- More concerned with the muscles which are kneaded, lifted or rolled.
- Circular, deep pressure through the muscles to release knots of tension.
- Patting, cupping or chopping movements to bring blood to the surface of the skin.

The massage should be neither painfully heavy nor irritatingly light and it should not hurt, although you should certainly be able to feel tight muscles being worked on. The therapist will feel the tension in your muscles to find out how much pressure to use, but it is also important for you to tell them if the pressure is too heavy or light. The therapist may use oil, lotion or talc.

Massage helps to eliminate toxins that have built up in the body and you may find that the first thing you want to do after a massage is to go to the toilet. It is also a good idea to drink plenty of water after a treatment to help flush out the toxins. After treatment you may feel sleepy and relaxed, so it is a good idea to plan to spend some time resting quietly after the massage to get the full benefit.

## Tips for making the most of your massage

- Before your treatment, you should have an empty stomach – do not eat too much for about two hours before your appointment.
- Give your therapist feedback – tell them if anything they are doing is uncomfortable, or if you want more attention paid to particular parts of your body.
- Remember, this is a time for your body to relax, so it is a good idea to focus on the massage itself, rather than use the time for social conversation. You may want to talk, or you may not. Do whatever feels right for you.
- Allow plenty of time for relaxation after the massage so that you can make the most of its soothing effect.

## *What is massage suitable for?*

Massage can be stimulating or sedating depending on the rate, rhythm and pressure of the strokes. It improves circulation, relaxes muscles and aids digestion. It also speeds up the elimination of waste products by stimulating the lymphatic system. Lymph is the milky white fluid that contains impurities and waste from the tissue cells.

On the emotional and psychological level it produces a feeling of ease and comfort. It is good for stress related problems such as high blood pressure, headaches and depression. The relaxing effect can also help to release tensions, calm the mind and induce a general feeling of well-being which can be useful in reducing or even eliminating the need for tranquillisers or sleeping pills.

Massage can have a profound effect on our emotions as we feel 'touched' at a deep level. This can result in an emotional release, improve our awareness and give us insight about our feelings. It can also help us to feel more aware of our bodies, which in turn can lead us to wanting to take better care of ourselves through diet and exercise.

Massage can be helpful for mechanical problems such as:

- Sprains, strains and other soft tissue problems such as tendititis
- Arthritis
- Back pain
- Carpel tunnel syndrome
- Repetitive strain injuries
- Sciatica
- Swelling around joints or injuries
- Impaired mobility and range of motion of joints

Most importantly, massage is enjoyable – and pleasure is therapeutic.

### ADVANTAGES OF THIS FORM OF TREATMENT

- It feels good to be touched.
- You do not have to feel ill in order to benefit from massage.
- It may be a form of preventative treatment as it helps the body to rid itself of toxins.

- Not everyone likes to be touched.

**SELF-TREATMENT**

Massage is one of the therapies you can use for self-treatment. Giving yourself a foot or hand massage can be very relaxing. But having someone else do it for you is so much more enjoyable.

# Biodynamic massage

From the words bio meaning life, and dynamic meaning movement, biodynamic massage is a form of massage which pays particular attention to tummy rumblings (peristaltic sounds). This therapy is based on the idea that there is an important link between our intestines and our unconscious – which is why we talk about 'gut reactions' and say, for example, 'I just knew it in my guts'.

## *History*

Biodynamic massage was developed by Norwegian physiotherapist and clinical psychologist Gerda Boysen in 1960. She had trained in both physical and psychological therapies and combined the two in a very powerful way. Working as a physiotherapist she noticed that when she massaged people, she could sometimes hear peristaltic sounds (tummy gurgling) when they were particularly relaxed. When she massaged people in ways that stimulated these gut reactions, patients often found that they were remembering long-forgotten events. Afterwards they described a sensation of peace, psychic cleanliness and 'lightness'. Their symptoms often disappeared.

Working as a psychologist, Gerda Boyson was aware of Sigmund Freud's ideas about the 'id canal'. She became interested in the work of Wilhelm Reich who was also convinced that the body must contain a physical aspect of the unconscious, and though he searched for it, he could not find it. Gerda Boysen found it in the form of the gut, the gastro-intestinal (GI) tract which made the gurgling sound. Her theory was that the intestines not only processed the physical waste products but also processed stress and unwanted thoughts and emotions. She found that she could help the body clear itself of blocked energy and could hear the result by listening to the change in peristaltic sounds.

Gerda Boysen set up a school in West London and has trained therapists who now work all over the world.

## What happens when you have a treatment?

Treatment starts with a short discussion of any health problems you may have had in the past as well as whatever may be currently troubling you. The therapist will ask you about what you want from the session and may invite you to make a contract, an agreement that you will have a particular number of sessions over a set length of time. This is very similar to what happens in counselling and you may experience biodynamic massage as a form of physical psychotherapy. However, you can 'contract' to have just a single session.

Exactly what form the massage depends on your needs. It may seem like an ordinary massage, with the only apparent differences being the use of talc rather than oil and the presence of a very long stethescope (which rests on your tummy so that the therapist can stay in touch with peristalsis). You may be massaged when you are stripped down to your underwear and covered with towels, or when you are fully clothed. It depends on you and what you want.

There is considerable emphasis on your emotional needs. You may remember incidents from the past, and the massage may help you release emotions such as anger or sadness along with any tension and stress.

## What is biodynamic massage suitable for?

It is suitable for any stress related ailment, especially if you are out of touch with your emotions. Examples of conditions that are particularly common in older people include:

- Arthritis
- Headache
- Backache

- Irritable bowel syndrome
- Digestive problems
- Sinus pain
- Colitis
- Anorexia and depression.

### ADVANTAGES OF THIS FORM OF TREATMENT

- It helps you get in touch with who you are at a gut level.
- It can help you release blocked emotions.

### DISADVANTAGES OF THIS FORM OF TREATMENT

- You may have problems finding a biodynamic massage therapist.
- You may want to keep your unconscious where it is – in the realm of the unconscious.

### SELF-TREATMENT

As with any form of massage, many of the techniques can be used on yourself.

## Help yourself exercises

These are simple, quick and effective ways of massaging yourself – even with your clothes on.

Stroke yourself, with your hands relaxed and open, in long motions, starting from the top of your head, down your shoulders and arms, down the front and back of your body, down your legs and right down to your feet. The quicker you do it the more energising it feels, the slower you do it, the more relaxing it feels.

If you want to enliven yourself try this sequence:
- Stroke yourself all over (as above).
- Tap all over your head, shoulders, arms, body, and legs using all five fingers.
- Knock on your shoulders, arms, body, and legs like knocking on a door.
- Stroke yourself all over (as above).

# Reflexology

A reflex is the involuntary response to nerve stimulation, and reflexology is a foot massage in which pressure on the foot has an effect on other parts of the body.

## *History of reflexology*

The ancient Egyptians used foot massage around 2500 BC. The tomb of the Egyptian doctor Ankmahor shows two darker skinned men 'working' on the feet of two men with lighter skin. The signs above the picture read:

*Patient*: 'Do not hurt me'

*Practitioner*: 'I shall act so you praise me'

Foot massage is also thought to have been practised in ancient China and India and amongst native American tribes. Traditional cultures believe the feet to be particularly important, as they help us to make contact with the earth.

In Europe a form of reflexology was known and practised as far back as the 14th century and in the 16th century, two books were published on 'zone therapy'. In London in 1898, Sir Henry Head discovered zones on the skin which became hypersensitive to pressure when an organ connected by nerves to this region were damaged. These were known as 'Head's zones' or 'zones of hyperalgesia'.

But it was the American Dr William Fitzgerald who made zone therapy famous. Dr Fitzgerald noticed that some patients experienced less pain than others, even when they had the same minor operations. He found that those who experienced very little pain were actually producing an anaesthetic effect by applying pressure to areas of their bodies – for example, by gripping the arm of the chair. Intrigued, he researched this while he was head physician at the Ear, Nose and Throat hospital in Hartford, Connecticut.

Dr Fitzgerald found that if pressure was applied to the fingers, it would create an anaesthetic effect on the hand, arm and shoulder, right up to the jaw, face, ear and nose. He applied pressure, using tight elastic bands on the middle section of each finger, or with small clamps which he placed on the fingertips. He successfully used this pressure technique to anaesthetise patients during minor surgical operations.

By using pressure on a specific part of the body, Dr Fitzgerald learned to predict which other parts of the body would be affected. He divided the body into zones. There are ten zones running the length of the body from the top of the head to the tips of the toes – each finger and toe falls within one zone. The zones are of equal width and extend right through the body from front to back. He believed that parts of the body found within a certain zone were linked to one another by the energy flow within the zone and could therefore affect one another.

Dr Fitzgerald and his colleague Dr Edwin Bowers tried to convince other doctors about their theory by applying pressure to the sceptical person's hand, then sticking a pin in the area of the face anaesthetised by the pressure. Although the demonstrations worked, most doctors remained unconvinced of the value of this therapy. In 1915 Dr Bowers wrote an article in *Everybody's Magazine* entitled 'Stop that toothache, squeeze your toe!' This was the first public description of the treatment they called 'zone therapy'. Two years later, in 1917, Fitzgerald and Bowers published the book *Zone Therapy*, which was largely ignored by the medical profession. However, Dr Joseph Riley was enthusiastic about the zone idea and his research assistant Eunice Ingham separated the work on the reflexes of the feet from zone therapy in general.

Eunice Ingham, known as the mother of modern reflexology, charted the feet in relation to the zones and their effects on the rest of the body. She drew up a map of the whole body that fitted neatly onto the feet – so for example, the tips of the toes relate to the brain and sinus, and the inside edge of the foot relates to the back. Her treatments were so effective that her reputation spread and she spent 30 years promoting her ideas through books, charts and seminars. Her two books *Stories the Feet can Tell* (published in 1938) and *Stories the Feet have Told* (published in 1951) were probably the first books to be written on the subject.

Doreen Bayly introduced reflexology into England in the 1960s. Danish-born Inge Dougens tried reflexology when she was told that she could not have children. She conceived after ten treatments and now has two sons. She was so impressed with the treatment that she trained as a reflexologist and wrote the book *The Art of Reflexology* in 1992. In the book she links reflexology with acupuncture. Dougens believes that reflexology works because it releases energy blockages in the meridiens, or energy channels in the body. The Metamorphic Technique also grew out of reflexology.

## The Metamorphic Technique

This method of featherlight foot massage was developed by the British naturopath and reflexologist Robert St John in the 1960s. He felt that the root of many long-standing, recurrent health problems was the result of difficulties during birth and immediately before birth, during the foetal stage in the womb. He also believed that there was a relationship between the foot and the body's develop-ment during the nine months foetal stage in the womb and that by lightly touching the inside of the foot and other reflex areas, these early problems can be resolved.

The technique uses extremely light touch on the feet, hands and head, and can be helpful for people who have been suffering from chronic health problems, or people who feel they are stuck in a rut and unable to make any changes in their life. It may also help peo-ple simply to come to terms with their situation.

## What happens when you have a treatment?

The reflexologist will ask about your medical history – what your current problems are, what diseases you have had in the past – and will also ask about any medicines you may be taking.

You will be invited to sit comfortably, either on a couch or a high back chair so you can sit up with your head and neck well support-ed. You will have to take off your socks, stockings or tights and it is helpful if you wear loose, comfortable clothes.

The reflexologist may start by cleaning your feet with witchhazel or some other form of cleanser. Then the reflexologist will use a gentle stroking movement to relax you before taking a detailed look at your feet. During this examination, reflexologists usually make notes of what they find, including details of:

- Temperature
- Muscle tone
- Tissue tone
- Skin condition
- Callouses, corns, and bunions and their position on the feet or toes.

These all provide the trained observer with valuable information about your state of health. For example, dry skin, cold, bluish or reddish feet may be signs of poor circulation. Feet that perspire may be a sign of a glandular imbalance. Tense feet may indicate tension in the body and limp feet may be a symptom of poor muscle tone. The position of corns and bunions etc. will alert the reflexologist to parts of your body which have problems. For example, a bunion may be a sign of a pancreas and thyroid imbalance. The general structure of the feet are also important. For example, if the second toe is longer than the big toe, this may be a sign of a weak digestive system.

Although the reflexologist can gather a vast amount of information about your health from simply looking at your feet, it is the treatment itself that is important. And this should feel wonderfully calming and comforting. Some people even find it exhilarating. It does not tickle because the quality of the touch is too firm.

Apart from the introductory stroking movements, most of the treatment is done by pressing the thumb firmly on particular points on the foot. This firm thumb pressure is directed at points which are as small as a pinhead and each point relates to different parts of the body. Pressure on different parts of the foot affects different parts of the body, so by the time both feet have been massaged your whole body will have felt the benefit.

The foot is always well supported and the pressure firm. You may experience different sensations in different parts of the feet which relate to your state of health in different parts of your body.

Congested areas will be sensitive – the more sensitive they are, the more congested the related areas will be. The sensations may range from the feeling of something sharp (like a piece of glass) being pressed into the foot, to a dull ache, discomfort, tightness or just firm pressure. If it hurts tell your reflexologist, who will then press more gently.

Reactions to reflexology vary from person to person, and from treatment to treatment. You may feel little or no tenderness at all during the first treatment, but your feet may become more sensitive with subsequent treatments. Even if you are not aware of very much happening during the reflexology session itself, when it is over you should feel light, tingly and thoroughly pampered.

The first treatment usually takes an hour, but follow-up treatments are often about 30–45 minutes. The longer you have had the problem, the longer it will take to cure, but you should see some signs of improvement fairly quickly. If reflexology is going to help with a health problem it should be obvious after three or four treatments. Reflexology does not work for everyone and if it has not helped after say four treatments, it probably never will.

Your reflexologist may suggest a course of treatment – perhaps twelve treatments once or twice a week. It may be best to have two sessions a week for a few weeks until there is an improvement.

## Reactions to reflexology treatment

On the whole, reactions immediately after a reflexology treatment are largely pleasant, and you will probably feel calm and relaxed or energised and rejuvenated. People often say that they sleep wonderfully well after a treatment and some people find that their skin tone and tissue texture have improved due to better circulation.

However, some people experience a healing reaction to treatment, so you may for example, need to go to the toilet more often as the kidneys and bowels flush out toxins. You may even find that you are producing more mucus and need to blow your nose more often.

Other signs of a healing reaction include:

- Increased perspiration and pimples
- Dizziness or nausea
- Increased discharge from the vagina in women
- Feverishness
- Tiredness.

It is helpful to drink plenty of pure water to help yourself through this cleansing process as quickly as possible. The healing reaction should not last for very long, and when it is over you should feel much, much better than you did before treatment started.

## What is reflexology suitable for?

Reflexogists say that this therapy is helpful for bringing people back into balance. It is particularly suitable for treating problems where the root of the problem is some form of blockage. It can help backaches, shoulder and neckaches, arthritis, gout, and digestive problems. It can also be a useful aid to rehabilitation after strokes.

Reflexology can help ease some of the symptoms of severe illnesses such as cancer. For example it can help to relieve pain, improve bladder and bowel control and stimulate the respiratory system. Reflexology can also be a very enjoyable, relaxing treatment that relieves stress.

### ADVANTAGES OF THIS FORM OF TREATMENT

- Simply being in calm, quiet surroundings where you are touched and have the undivided attention of one other person relieves stress and is relaxing and soothing. It's a pleasant, enjoyable way of nurturing and taking care of yourself.
- Reflexology has similar stress relieving benefits to a full body massage, without the need to get undressed or be touched all over.

### DISADVANTAGES OF THIS FORM OF TREATMENT

- Reflexology does not suit everybody – you may not enjoy the experience of having your feet touched. You may also find that although it is pleasant enough, it does not actually cure any of your health problems. On the other hand, it may have a profoundly healing effect, but it may stir things up and it may have a strong, cleansing effect on your body.

- Anyone can call themselves a reflexologist after little or no training, so it is important to go to an experienced, well-qualified therapist.
- Reflexology should be avoided on parts of your foot where there are varicose veins as they can be damaged by treatment. If you have an infection such as athlete's foot, it is not a good idea to have reflexology as the infection may spread.

#### SELF-TREATMENT

Although it is perfectly possible to work on the reflexes of your own feet, this is not nearly as enjoyable as having someone else do it for you.

## Resources

*The Art of Reflexology* by Inge Dougans with Suzanne Ellis, Element Books, 1992

# Acupressure

Popularly known as 'acupuncture without the needles', acupressure uses massage points on the energy channels or meridians.

## History of acupressure

We instinctively press our forehead when we have a headache, and acupressure is probably one of the oldest aspects of traditional Chinese medicine, pre-dating acupuncture.

A form of massage was used in ancient China which was known as *anmo*, and changed its name slightly when it was adopted by the Japanese who called it *anma* or *do-in-anka*. The therapy included exercises, diet, and meditation as well as massage and manipulation. It became a profession associated with blind people who were particularly skilled at this form of massage which eventually developed into acupressure.

Acupressure is still widely used by Japanese families as a form of first aid for pain relief as well as preventative medicine. Regular acupressure improves vitality by keeping the energy channels flowing free (blockages are thought to cause disease). The therapy has many forms, including Jin Shin Do and Shin Tao, which vary in the combination of pressure points and the amount of pressure used. In Britain, shiatsu is the most popular form of acupressure (see the following section).

The basic idea behind acupressure – that firm pressure on particular points can be healing – has also been used by a number of Western therapies such as:

- Reflexology
- C-bands for travel sickness
- Kinesiology
- Massage.

## What happens when you have a treatment?

You may be asked for your medical details in the usual way. The therapist may also use traditional Chinese medicine diagnostic techniques such as feeling your pulses and looking at your tongue to see which imbalances need to be corrected.

It is a good idea to wear loose, comfortable clothes for the treatment as you will be fully clothed when it is carried out. You will usually be asked to lie on a firm mattress or mat on the floor, although some therapists use a table.

There are different forms of acupressure and every therapist has their own way of working and will apply pressure in different ways. They may use thumbs, fingers, palms, knees, elbows, even feet. The point may be tender and it may hurt or you may feel a sudden chill, but these kind of symptoms only last a couple of seconds, just while the point is being pressed.

Therapists may suggest that you practise yoga-like exercises which stretch the meridians, and they may show you pressure points which you can use yourself to relieve your symptoms. They may also suggest changes in your diet which are based on traditional Chinese medicine principles (see the section on TCM in Chapter 4).

A session usually lasts for 30 minutes to an hour. If you are being treated for a particular problem, it is a good idea to go weekly, or you can go when you feel like it for a tune up as a preventative measure.

## What is acupressure suitable for?

Acupressure helps to unblock stagnant energy and so it can be helpful for pain relief as well as a form of preventative medicine. In relation to diseases which are common in older people, it is particularly helpful for arthritis, asthma, back pain, circulation problems, depression, digestive problems, insomnia, migraine and tension.

### PAIN RELIEF

Like acupuncture, acupressure releases healing energy along the meridians which helps to relieve pain and discomfort.

### PREVENTION

Working on acupressure points eases muscular tension and releases tensions and toxins before they develop into disease. The aim is to release toxins before they cause damage to internal organs.

### ADVANTAGES OF THIS FORM OF TREATMENT

● Acupressure is a gentle therapy which allows the whole body to be treated and touched while you stay fully clothed.

### DISADVANTAGES OF THIS FORM OF TREATMENT

● Not everyone enjoys the sensations of the acupressure points being pressed.

### SELF-TREATMENT

This therapy is safe to use on yourself, and the acupressure practitioner will probably encourage you to help yourself.

## Self-help acupressure

■ For headache, toothache, cramps and constipation, squeeze the web of flesh between the thumb and index finger for about five minutes, the pressure should be towards the index finger.
■ For nausea such as travel sickness or anxiety, press your thumb on the point about two inches (50mm) from the wrist for five to ten minutes.

# Shiatsu

Literally translated from Japanese as finger pressure, shiatsu combines ancient forms of oriental massage with modern Western techniques of both Swedish massage and manipulation.

## History of shiatsu

While shiatsu is a relatively modern therapy, it can trace its roots to traditional Chinese medicine which was introduced into Japan more than 1000 years ago. At the time, massage was used as a therapy alongside acupuncture and herbal medicine, but the therapeutic use of massage went into decline in the 18th and 19th centuries when it was mainly used for pleasure and comfort.

Tokujuro Namikoshi developed shiatsu after treating his mother's rheumatism by massage, and found that firm pressure on certain points relieved her pain.

## Shiatsu – key dates

| | |
|---|---|
| 1925 | Namikoshi opened the Shiatsu Institute of Therapy |
| 1940 | Japan Shiatsu Institute opened (now known as the Japan Shiatsu School) |
| 1964 | Shiatsu officially recognised by the Japanese government |

Today, shiatsu has helped massage to regain its therapeutic status in Japan, where it is practised alongside acupuncture and herbalism. Apart from professional shiatsu therapists, nearly everyone in Japan practises some form of shiatsu or massage, if only to relieve stress and tension in the neck and shoulders.

Shiatsu schools have opened in England and all over the world.

## What happens when you have a treatment?

Wear loose comfortable clothes for your treatment, which will usually be carried out on a mat on the floor.

Some therapists will ask for your medical details in the usual way, others prefer to let your body do the talking. The session may start with the practitioner using traditional Chinese medicine diagnosis, which may take the form of the practitioner lightly touching your belly, or they may take your pulse and look at your tongue.

Shiatsu therapists' own movements are an important part of the therapy, and they will usually begin by kneeling beside you, and then moving around, using their body weight, breathing patterns and even their own energy (or chi) as well as their hands. Pressure may be applied to your sacrum, and different techniques will be used to stretch out the spine such as lifting, placing in different positions and even gentle pulling.

Although shiatsu means 'finger pressure', practitioners also use palms, elbows, knees and even their bare feet. The pressure may vary from light to quite firm and may include rubbing, kneading, brushing and pummelling, almost like an ordinary massage. Part of the session may include light holding techniques and gentle stretches and manipulation techniques are used which help to release blocked energy and stimulate blood flow.

Generally the practitioner works on the whole of the body. The session should not be painful, but if you experience any discomfort you should tell your practitioner.

You may be given advice about your lifestyle and diet and you may be given some simple exercises to do at home to speed up the recovery process and help you to be independent.

Sessions last from 40–60 minutes although the first session may be slightly longer.

To get the most out of the treatment you will be encouraged to close your eyes and focus on what you feel.

The treatment is very relaxing and after a session your body should feel freer and looser and you may have a greater sense of serenity, wholeness and well-being. You may feel you have more energy or you may be tired and need to sleep.

After the session, it is a good idea to go home and rest for a couple of hours and not do anything stressful so that you can make the most of the treatment. You should feel some immediate benefits, but if you are uncomfortable, contact your practitioner.

You may want weekly treatments at first, then fortnightly and monthly, but it is a good idea to discuss this with your practitioner so that you can both decide what is best for you.

## What is shiatsu suitable for?

The main value of shiatsu is as a form of preventative medicine to maintain health and stamina. It unblocks blocked energy and balances energy so that not too much energy is focused in one area. Relating particularly to diseases which are common in older people, shiatsu is particularly helpful for arthritis, digestive problems, circulation problems, back problems, headaches and depression.

### ADVANTAGES OF THIS FORM OF TREATMENT

- It works well with other forms of treatment.
- It is done while you are fully clothed.
- It is gentle and enables your whole body to be touched.
- It can be adapted to suit you. For example, if you are frail or disabled then less manipulation can be used.

### DISADVANTAGES OF THIS FORM OF TREATMENT

- Not everyone likes to be touched.

### SELF-TREATMENT

You may be given some shiatsu techniques to practise on your own.

# Kinesiology

Pronounced kin-easy-ology, the name of this therapy comes from the Greek words *kinesis* meaning motion and *logos* meaning to study. Literally, it is 'the study of movement'. It uses muscle testing for diagnosis and treatment.

## History of kinesiology

Kinesiology was developed in the mid-1960s by an American doctor of chiropractic, George Goodheart. At the time, most chiropractors worked mainly with the bones, although they also gave nutritional and lifestyle advice. But Goodheart started to work with the muscles as well. He found that strengthening the muscles could have a dramatic effect on his clients' health. For example, if someone was suffering from indigestion, Goodheart found that working with one of the pectoral muscles at the top of the chest (*pectoralis major clavicular*) would strengthen the stomach and ease the indigestion.

Goodheart discovered that there were many different ways of strengthening weak muscles, including working with nutrition and acupressure points. He developed his ideas into a complete system which he called *Applied Kinesiology* which is taught only to chiropractors and other medical professionals. One of his students, chiropractor John Thie started to teach his patients some simple exercises and massage points to encourage them to work on themselves in between treatments. This helped them to recover more quickly. Thie simplified normal kinesiology and taught it to people who had no medical background. He called it *'Touch for Health'*. Using these new techniques, ordinary people found that they could use kinesiology for a wide range of problems. They developed their own forms of kinesiology such as Health Kinesiology, Creative Kinesiology, Educational Kinesiology etc.

In Britain over the past decade the different forms of kinesiology have amalagmated to form a single professional body which is known as the Kinesiology Federation.

## What happens during a consultation?

After asking about your medical history and the things you want to change, the kinesiologist will also ask about what you want to achieve during the course of treatment and discuss the history of any problems you want to work on.

You will be invited to lie down on a couch, fully clothed. The kinesiologist will then test your muscles by asking you to put an arm or leg into a particular position and hold it steady. The kinesiologist then presses gently for a few seconds to find out how well you can resist this gentle pressure. If the muscle does not respond normally, the practitioner makes a series of other muscle tests to find out why.

Muscle testing can help the kinesiologist to find out about a wide range of problems which may need treating. These may include mis-aligned bones, organs and glands which are not functioning well, emotional stresses that need diffusing, nutritional needs, allergies, as well as energetic and electrical disturbances.

The muscle testing enables the kinesiologist to find out:

- Which problems need to be addressed – and in what order.
- What needs to be done to solve the problems – and in what order.
- Whether the treatment has been successful.

Kinesiologists use a wide range of therapies including:

- Chiropractic
- Massage
- Acupressure
- Vitamins and mineral supplements
- Emotional release
- Allergy desensitisation
- Bach flower remedies.

The corrections and treatments are usually painless and give imme-diate results. It is a good idea to have weekly treatments for a few weeks – then monthly until you are well enough to need a session just every now and again to help you stay healthy.

Each treatment lasts for about an hour. You will probably find that it is very relaxing and you should feel clearer and lighter afterwards, although you may feel tired or sleepy. It is a good idea to rest fol-lowing treatments.

## What is kinesiology suitable for?

Kinesiology is concerned with balance, and in that balancing process it can be used to keep you healthy or to treat a wide variety of ail-ments. Referring particularly to diseases which are common in older people, such ailments include backache, sciatica, headaches, migraine, stiff joints, low energy, and depression.

## ADVANTAGES OF THIS FORM OF TREATMENT

- Kinesiology is not restricted to any one form of treatment, but uses the most appropriate means of strengthening your muscles (and your whole body).
- It is possible to use a surrogate. If you are too ill or frail to be tested, someone else can hold your hand and be tested as if they were you.

## DISADVANTAGES OF THIS FORM OF TREATMENT

- Not everyone likes to be touched or have their muscles tested.

Kinesiology is an unusual therapy. It challenges people's assumptions that if something is wrong physically, then the solution is automatically physical. If you go to a kinesiologist about a backache, there is really no telling what they will use to make it better – it can be anything from acupressure to emotional stress release, or a combination of several therapies.

## SELF-TREATMENT

Although you can use muscle testing in the family, you can't really do it on your own. However, there are some self-help techniques which kinesiologists sometimes recommend, as shown in the box.

## Emotional stress release

This exercise uses the points which are like bumps halfway between the middle of your eyebrows and your hairline (or where your hairline used to be).

- Close your eyes and place your fingertips lightly over these points.
- Think about whatever is troubling you.
- Experience the problem by being as aware of it as clearly as you possibly can by thinking about what it feels like, sounds like, even what it smells like.
- Keep thinking about the problem.

■ When it gets difficult to focus on the issue, release your fingertips, open your eyes and think again about the situation and how you feel about it now.

This process can take one to ten minutes and you may feel your head pulsing erratically at first.

**Stimulate the lymphatic system and the immune system**
You can stimulate the lymphatic system and the immune system by waking up the thymus gland. Use all five fingers of one hand, tap under the upper breast bone in the centre of the chest for about 20 seconds.

## Resources

*Thorsons Introductory Guide to Kinesiology* by Maggie La Tourelle with Anthea Courtnay, Thorsons, 1992

*Kinesiology* by Ann Holdway, Element, 1995

# Zero balancing

This therapy involves a way of being touched at bone level which brings balance, healing and relaxation. Zero balancing pays particular attention to the parts of the skeleton that can be considered as 'shock absorbers'.

## Joints as shock absorbers

Within the skeletal system there are several joints which have a minimal range of motion and whose main function is related to the transmission of energetic forces. These joints, such as the sacroiliac joint, are known as 'foundation joints' and are a major focus of zero balancing. When such joints become compressed, the body tends to compensate in a way that may have widespread effects. These compensations may impede function and set up unconscious tensions that lead to a reduction in our vitality and can limit our potential for health.

## History of zero balancing

Zero balancing was developed by Dr Fritz Smith who trained as a doctor, osteopath and acupuncturist. He practised meditation and yoga in his search for a way of combining Western knowledge of our physical structure with eastern understanding of how energy moves in the body. Affectionately called 'Zee Bee', zero balancing came together in its current form when Fritz Smith was in England studying acupuncture in the mid-1970s, and many of the first people he taught were acupuncturists. In 1986, he published the book *Inner Bridges*, which goes into detail of how he developed zero balancing.

At the moment, training is restricted to therapists who have already qualified in another form of medicine such as doctors, acupuncturists, osteopaths, massage therapists, counsellors and physiotherapists. They use zero balancing to enhance existing skills as well as a system in its own right.

## What happens when you have a treatment?

The zero balancer may start by asking you a few questions about how you are feeling and about any problems you may be having. You will be invited to sit on a massage couch (fully clothed). The zero balancer will then lift up one of your arms and move it in a gentle circle, and then repeat the process with the other arm. You will then be asked to move from one side and then another, while the practitioner supports your lower back. This is done partly to help the zero balancer to get to know the way your body moves, and partly to let your body know how the practitioner's hands feel. You will then be invited to lie on the couch.

The session itself will follow several, seamless stages. The zero balancer will:

- Assess how your body feels and moves – thereby allowing you to become aware of your body, and how it feels and moves.
- Use finger pressure and held stretches (called fulcrums), which allows your body to relax.
- Assess how your body has changed. This also gives you an awareness of your body and how it might have changed.

The touch zero balancers use is very clear. There is a feeling that your bones are being invited to relax, to adjust themselves into the most comfortable position. Zero balancers work with 'the shock absorbers of the body' – the bones and joints, such as those of the spine, which don't move very much. The same joints tend to get compressed with the force of gravity, stress, strain and accidents. The zero balancer invites these tightly compressed bones to release by gently lifting up the bones on either side. For example, in order to release the spine, the zero balancer creates a fulcrum by touching the ribs on either side of the spine.

You may feel your back being gently lifted and returned to its original position, except it is not quite in the same position, it may feel different in some way, you may feel longer, lighter, easier and more relaxed. Your legs and hips, neck and head will be moved and held in a similar way.

Zero balancing helps you to get in touch with yourself – your body isn't told what it should, or shouldn't be doing. The effect is similar to meditation, helping you to feel deeply relaxed and peaceful. The zero balancer will feel what is happening to your bones with their fingertips and see the way your energy is shifting, by noticing such signals as eyelids fluttering, yawning, tummy rumbles etc. In the words of Fritz Smith 'Our deepest nature is held in our bone and when you touch someone this way they certainly know about it, it is very profound' (quoted by Susan Clark in *The Times*, September 28, 1999).

Responses to zero balancing vary from person to person and from session to session, so that after a session you may feel light and elated, or you may be aware of feeling more rooted and grounded. During the session you may be aware of old memories from childhood, or receive insights about what is happening in your life at the moment as part of the dialogue between you and your body. When the session is finished, you will be encouraged to walk up and down the room for a few times. This is to help you settle and get used to your newly balanced body.

A zero balancing session lasts between 20 and 40 minutes.

## What is zero balancing suitable for?

Zero balancing is a method of helping you to get in touch with yourself and your body. It is a method of amplifying wellness rather than treating illness. In that process it has been known to help many things, including poor sleep patterns, restricted movements, and lack of vitality. It can also be helpful for such physical complaints as backache, aching joints, sciatica, headache and migraines.

Because the bones are such a fundamental part of ourselves, zero balancing can help us get in touch with our own structure, our own way of dealing with things. This can be helpful on an emotional and psychological level, particularly if you are going through a big change in your life, suffering from stress, bereavement or generally feeling at a loss with what to do with your life.

### ADVANTAGES OF THIS FORM OF TREATMENT

- It is undemanding and relaxing.
- It helps you explore where you are, where you have been, and where you could be through awareness of your body, but without having to do anything more than lie there and pay attention.
- It does not force the body to make changes it is not ready for.

### DISADVANTAGES OF THIS FORM OF TREATMENT

- It is not a treatment for sick people, although it may be very helpful with specific complaints.
- There are certain complaints that do not respond to zero balancing, but these depend very much on the individual and the experience of the therapist.

### SELF-TREATMENT

Zero balancing is not suitable for self-treatment.

## Resources

*Inner Bridges* by Fritz Smith, Humanics New Age, 1986

*Zero Balancing* by John Hamwee, Frances Lincoln, 2000

'Zero balancing – a therapy to harmonise mind and body'. Susan Clark, *The Times*, September 28, 2000.

# 6
# Energy Therapies

## Introduction

Look at happy-go-lucky toddlers running around, falling over, picking themselves up again, crying one minute and laughing the next. They have plenty of free flowing energy which is why they are constantly on the move. As we get older, it takes longer to pick ourselves up when we fall. It takes more to make us laugh or cry. Everything takes slightly longer. It is part of the growing up process – it is also part of the growing older process.

Energy medicine can help us make the most of the energy that we have, release blocks to our energy flowing freely and help us to contact the source of infinite energy.

We all instinctively understand energy. We take it for granted when we've got plenty of it and complain about it when we don't have enough. We talk about energy as if we can measure it, and like the wind we recognise where it is, even if we can't see it.

'He's bubbling with energy and enthusiasm'.
'She's got so much energy, I don't know how she does it'.
'He looks drained, all his energy seems to have gone'.
'Sorry, I can't do that today, I've got no energy'.

According to the *Collins Pocket Dictionary*, energy means forcefulness, the capacity to do work and overcome resistance, capacity for intense activity, vigour, intensity or vitality of action or expression.

The therapies in this section are all concerned with our energy bodies, just as the therapies in the physical therapies section are concerned with our physical bodies. We react to stress and trauma with our physical bodies becoming tense, painful and out of alignment, our energy bodies react slightly differently – although the effect is the same.

Servicing our physical bodies helps the mechanical parts of ourselves to move as smoothly as possible with the minimum of wear and tear. The same is true of our energy bodies. Our energy bodies can get just as stressed and out of alignment as our physical bodies and they need just as much attention if we are going to 'run' smoothly.

With the therapies in this section, the starting point is energy, although they affect all the other parts of ourselves: our physical, mental, emotional, and spiritual selves.

Energy medicine usually makes us feel better from the inside out – we feel better mentally, emotionally and spiritually before our physical complaints clear up. Sometimes there is a dramatic improvement, but this is rare, and a more gradual, subtle change is more likely. Sometimes the change is so subtle, we may even forget what was wrong with us in the first place.

The energy therapies include:

- **Acupuncture** The acupuncturist releases blocked energy channels and stimulates areas which are weak with very fine needles. These needles adjust the energy in your meridians or energy channels. Again the results can be quite dramatic or they can be subtle and it may take a few sessions before you feel the benefit.
- **Healing** Healers channel divine or universal healing energy which works with your own healing energy. The way they do this is by holding their hands lightly on or near your body, which is very relaxing and pleasant. It is perfectly possible to have a miraculous healing experience but, by their nature, miracles are rare. It is much more likely that you will feel pleasantly relaxed and cherished after a healing session and experience a gradual improvement in your symptoms over several sessions. You may also gain some emotional or spiritual understanding of what is happening in your life.
- **Homeopathy** The treatment is the energy in a little white pill which works with your own healing energy. The effect can be dramatic – or a complete waste of time if the homeopath has not

found the right remedy. When it works well, it can feel as if every aspect of your being has shifted. It can also work more slowly and subtly, particularly if you have had the complaint for some time.

## Energy exercise

This exercise is designed to help you feel your own energy.

■ Sit in a comfortable position with your back upright, feet flat on the floor. Now close your eyes and take a couple of deep breaths.

■ Imagine you have got a ball between your hands, and play with this imaginary ball, feeling it getting larger and smaller.

■ Now feel the space between your hands, it probably feels different to the space that is on the back of your hands.

■ Play with your hands, making the imaginary ball get bigger and smaller, bringing your hands closer together and then further apart. You will probably feel that your hands are meeting a subtle form of resistance. This may be heat or coldness or a feeling of denseness. Different people experience different things, it can be quite subtle or not so subtle.

■ Bring your hands out as wide as you can and then bring them in closer and closer together until you feel some resistance, a feeling of denseness or heat. Notice how far apart your hands are.

Different people feel this energy in different ways, but it is a good way to experience your own energy field – it gives you an idea of what we're talking about in this section of the book, when we talk about energy.

## Acupuncture

The word acupuncture means 'to prick with a needle'. It is an ancient Chinese therapy which is based on the idea that illnesses are caused by energy imbalances which can be cured by sticking needles into the skin at particular points.

## *History of acupuncture*

According to Chinese legend, acupuncture grew out of the observation that soldiers who survived arrow wounds sometimes also recovered from other long-standing complaints.

Acupuncture is thought to be 4,500 years old as sharp instruments which could be used for puncturing skin have been found in archeological digs from the stone age onwards. Needles have been found in the form of splinters of sharp stone, pottery, bone, wood, iron and bronze. In more recent times, gold and silver needles were used and today, they are usually made from stainless steel.

Over the centuries various rulers have tried unsuccessfully to ban acupuncture in China and introduce Western medicine. However, acupuncture and other forms of traditional Chinese medicine were encouraged by Mao Tse Tung during the Red Revolution because so few doctors were trained in Western medicine and drugs and medical equipment were scarce. In modern China, acupuncture is used alongside Western medicine. Perhaps the most dramatic example of this is when acupuncture is used as the anaesthetic during surgery. Acupuncture is such a popular form of treatment that it is as easy to buy acupuncture needles in China as it is to buy aspirin in England. Acupuncture is used to treat anything and everything, hence the Chinese expression: 'A single needle can treat 10,000 maladies'.

British doctors have used acupuncture since the early 19th century when it was introduced into Europe by Jesuit missionaries returning from China. In 1823, the first edition of the medical journal *The Lancet* carried a detailed report of the successful use of acupuncture in treating rheumatism.

## Acupuncture through the ages

| | |
|---|---|
| 400BC | First acupuncture textbook, *The Yellow Emperor's Classic of Internal Medicine* (Nei Ching Si Wem). |
| 400BC | The first recorded acupuncture success story. A doctor called Pein Chueh used it to revive a patient who was in a coma. |
| 250AD to 600AD | Acupuncture developed rapidly in China, and books and coloured charts describing the channels and points for the treatment of various conditions appeared. |
| 960AD | First recorded use of moxibustion. The word moxibustion derives from the Japanese word mokusa meaning burning herb. Instead of pricking the skin with a needle, common mugwort is burned close to the skin. This form of acupuncture is still used today. |
| 1644 onwards | Acupuncture was brought to Europe by Jesuit missionaries returning from China. It was first introduced to Germany in the 17th century, and then into France in the middle of the 19th century. |
| Early 19th century | Acupuncture first used by British doctors. |
| 1823 | The first edition of the medical journal *The Lancet* contains a detailed report of the successful use of acupuncture in treating rheumatism. |
| 1929 | The rulers of the Ching dynasty tried to ban acupuncture, but failed to suppress it completely. |
| 1934–5 | Mao Tse Tung used acupuncture and other forms of traditional medicine to keep his soldiers healthy during his rise to power. |
| 1949 | Establishment of the People's Republic of China and the resurgence of interest in acupuncture, particularly in combining its use with Western medicine. |

## What happens when you have a treatment?

### THE DIAGNOSIS

The acupuncturist will ask you a lot of questions about your health. Apart from the usual questions about your medical history, you will also be asked about your whole way of life and details about your complaint. Questions may include:

- What do you like to eat and drink?
- How well do you sleep?
- Does it hurt when you move?
- Is it worse in the mornings?
- What else makes it worse?
- What makes it better?

To complete the diagnosis, the acupuncturist will also ask to look at your tongue and feel your pulses. The tongue can tell an acupuncturist a great deal about what is happening inside the body. For example, a yellow coating on the tongue shows that there is a problem with too much heat, while a white coating suggests a lot of moisture. The acupuncturist will gather other clues about your condition by looking at the way you stand and sit, the shape and colour of your face, and even the way you smell.

According to traditional Chinese medicine (TCM) there are twelve meridians or energy pathways. They run in lines throughout your body, and it is these meridians that acupuncturists feel when they take your pulses (six meridians on the left wrist, six meridians on the right wrist). Some of the meridians are concerned with particular organs:

- The heart
- The small intestine
- The gallbladder
- The kidney
- The liver
- The lungs
- The colon
- The stomach.

Although these meridians are named after organs, they refer to the energy of the organ and not just the organ itself. For example, the kidney meridian is concerned with:

- Ears
- Eyes
- Bones
- Bone marrow
- Saliva
- Head hair
- Genitals
- Urethra
- Anus.

Since the adrenal glands are situated on top of the kidneys and are responsible for the fight or flight response, it is not surprising that the kidney meridian is associated with fear. If you feel jumpy, agitated, anxious or fearful, the acupuncturist may find that there is a problem with the kidney meridian.

Apart from deciding which meridian is out of balance, the acupuncturist also has to decide what needs to be done to correct the imbalance. They will decide on exactly which points on the meridians to insert the needles – originally there were 365 points to choose from, but so many more have been discovered that the modern acupuncturist has a choice of over 2,000. The needles unblock, increase or decrease the flow of energy called Chi (pronounced chee) through the meridians.

In TCM, there is a saying: 'Anything can come from anything'. When acupuncturists make a diagnosis, they don't name the disease but the source of the imbalance in the energy of the person. The questions to be answered are:

- What is the state of this person's chi?
- What has happened to disrupt the flow?
- What are the internal strengths that can be used to promote self healing?

Answering these kind of questions will help the practitioner decide which acupuncture points to use. For example, if someone has high blood pressure, it could be that the person has too much energy in the liver meridian and too little in the kidney meridian. The treatment may be to calm the liver point known as supreme rushing and to boost the kidney point which is called greater mountain stream.

## THE TREATMENT

The associations most people have with needles may cause anxieties about whether acupuncture will hurt. Actually, it doesn't – or rather shouldn't – hurt much, if at all.

The needles are usually very fine, so it doesn't feel like an injection or a blood test, in fact some people barely feel them at all, others experience them as a light prick. If the needles do hurt, tell your acupuncturist who will either adjust the way the needle is resting or take it out and try again. Once the needles are in, they shouldn't hurt, although you may be aware of them being in place.

The acupuncturist may press the point before inserting the needle. This slight pressure may feel sharp, or just slightly tense. You may be asked to breathe in just before the needle is inserted, and breathe out when the needle is actually inserted.

You will be lying down during the treatment and may find this very relaxing, particularly if you have been feeling tense or agitated beforehand. After the treatment, you may feel invigorated, sleepy, or just unaware of any reaction. But however you feel it is a good idea to have a rest as soon as possible after the session, to take full advantage of the treatment. People react in several different ways to an acupuncture session — you may even feel worse, or you may feel extremely tired. If you feel tired, it means that your body is concentrating its energy on the healing process.

If your symptoms are worse after an acupuncture treatment it may be that your body is going through a period of detoxification. This clearing out process may cause a temporary, mild fever, sweating, or skin disorders. These are usually good signs and when these symptoms pass, you usually feel much better than before the treatment as your vital force is no longer hampered by whatever was poisoning your system. Whatever reaction you have to the treatment though, you should tell your acupuncturist about it on your next visit. This will help them to understand the way your energy works, and enable them to fine tune your treatment.

The first few treatments will probably be only a week or two apart but, as your health improves, there will be increasing gaps between visits. You may need to go every three or four weeks or, if you are fairly healthy, the acupuncturist may only want to see you four times a year to help your energy change and adapt with the seasons.

The first consultation lasts an hour or more. Follow-up treatments are slightly shorter.

## What is acupuncture suitable for?

Whether acupuncture can help you depends on several factors:

- The skill of the acupuncturist – the more experienced the therapist the more likely they are to make an accurate diagnosis and treatment.
- The state of your vital force – the greater your vital force or chi, the easier it is for acupuncture to work.
- Your own behaviour and environment – the healthier your diet and lifestyle, the easier it is for acupuncture to help you.
- The nature of the complaint itself and how long you have had it – the longer you have suffered from the complaint, the harder it is to treat.

The general rule with acupuncture and most of the natural therapies is that the sooner a complaint is dealt with, the better the chances of a cure. Unfortunately, most people only turn to acupuncture when all else has failed, but it is still well worthwhile trying acupuncture for chronic complaints.

Acupuncture's effectiveness relies on its ability to improve the flow of chi in the body. Acupuncture can only harness the energy that is there, so the less chi or energy a person has, the harder it is to treat. Children respond very quickly to acupuncture because they have plenty of energy. Illness and age reduce the amount of energy available, so the response to acupuncture may be slow or even non-existent. In such circumstances, other forms of TCM such as herbs may be used to boost a person's chi, thus making acupuncture more effective.

The acupuncturist may suggest other changes to boost your energy, such as having more rest and eating more vegetables. To some extent the ability of acupuncture to help you is limited by your ability to help yourself. Acupuncture won't help bruises heal if you keep bashing your head against a brick wall! Similarly, neither acupuncture nor any other therapy will be able to cure chest problems if you carry on smoking, or diabetes if you overeat. There are also less obvious examples where acupuncture can help you only if you help yourself. For example, if your system is seriously depleted, all the acupuncture in the world won't help if you keep adding to the problem by working too much, or resting too little.

Cancer provides an example of where acupuncture can be helpful in different ways, at various stages of the disease. Acupuncture used at an early stage may slow down the development of the growth. If the cancer has reached a stage where there has been severe damage to the organ concerned, surgery may be necessary, but acupuncture can be used to help recovery after the operation. It can also be useful when people have terminal cancer, helping both to control the pain and to calm the spirit.

Parkinson's disease can be helped with acupuncture, but most people with Parkinson's only try acupuncture when the disease is at a relatively late stage which makes treatment difficult. Even so, acupuncture may reduce the amount of medication that is needed and slow down the process of the disease. It's particularly suitable for people who can't take the usual drug (dopamine) as acupuncture can calm the tremors and ease the stiffness associated with the disease. In Alzheimer's disease too, people tend to turn to acupuncture at a late stage. Unfortunately by the time symptoms appear, there has already been considerable degeneration and disruption to the brain cells and the best that acupuncture can hope to achieve is a slowing down of the degenerative process.

Acupuncture can be surprisingly helpful for emotional or spiritual problems. You may have noticed yourself that there are days when you feel heavy and depressed and then something mysteriously shifts and your mood changes – this shows that the chi is moving smoothly again. Acupuncture can help depression by improving the flow of chi. It can also be helpful for sleeping difficulties such as insomnia.

Here the Chinese understanding is that we can only sleep well when our 'shen', or spirit, is at peace, resting safely in our hearts. Acupuncture can be used to encourage the shen to return to its natural resting place. Pent up feelings of grief and despair can also be released with the help of acupuncture.

Arthritis is particularly well suited to acupuncture treatment. While it cannot rejuvenate deformed joints, it can increase mobility and relieve pain.

Other problems which may respond well to acupuncture include:

- Hypertension
- Heart disease
- Diabetes
- Rehabilitation after strokes
- Eye problems. Acupuncture is particularly helpful for optic atrophy (the main cause of blindness in older people) and neuritis. It can also help with cataracts if treatment starts early enough.

### ADVANTAGES OF ACUPUNCTURE

- Acupuncture is relatively cheap compared to Western medicine.
- This is a gentle, effective treatment with no side-effects.
- It can be used with good results in conjunction with Western medicine.
- It also provides a non-invasive, inexpensive method of diagnosis.

### DISADVANTAGES OF ACUPUNCTURE

- Acupuncture is only as effective as the practitioner.
- It cannot renew damaged parts of the body (such as hips, hearts etc.)
- Effective symptom relief can mask serious problems such as cancer.
- It is not suitable for emergency treatment (such as heart attacks) in the UK, simply because acupuncturists don't work in hospitals.
- Not everyone can cope with the idea of the needles.

SELF-TREATMENT

Acupuncture is not suitable for the do-it-yourself approach, but an acupuncturist may suggest ways in which you can help yourself through other forms of TCM (see the section on Traditional Chinese Medicine in Chapter 4).

## Resources

*The Complete Book of Energy Medicine*, by Dr Helen Dziemidko. Gaia, 1999

# Spiritual healing

Spiritual healing is the process where the practitioner focuses healing energy and the person who receives this energy can use it to make themselves healthy again. Some people call it the power of prayer or the laying on of hands. It refers to any form of healing where the healing energy comes from the Divine, which is whatever you understand as the source of all energy.

## History of spiritual healing

Spiritual healing is as old as humankind. Mothers who have looked after their sick children know what it is like to ask for help and healing from a source that is greater than ourselves. Traditional cultures and ancient tribes all have their own versions of healers, medicine men and wise ones whose role is to bring healing to the people, linking the physical, mortal world, to the immortal, spiritual world.

The oldest records we have on healing dates back to Hippocrates who wrote:

It is believed by experienced doctors that the heat which oozes out of the hand, on being applied to the sick is highly salutary. It has often appeared while I have been soothing my patients as if there was a singular property in my hands to pull and draw away from the affected parts aches and diverse impurities by laying my hand upon the place and by extending my fingers towards it. Thus it is known to some of the learned that health may be implanted in the sick by certain gestures, and by contact, as some diseases may be communicated from one to another.

Many ancient religions believed that disease is a message from the gods and priests were also healers. But the Christian church started to separate healing from preaching and in the 13th century a papal decree forbade priests to practise surgery, dissect bodies or even study anatomy.

This separation gave healing a bad name, and healers were persecuted. Only kings and queens were allowed to heal, as it seemed that the royal touch cured people with tuberculosis of the skin. But even this form of healing died out and the last royal healer in Britain was Queen Anne who healed Dr Johnson in 1712 when he was two and a half.

In 1905 three Anglican priests formed the Guild of Health as part of their crusade to reawaken the church's wider responsibly for health and healing. The idea was slow in starting and it was only towards the end of the 20th century that Christian churches once again involved themselves with spiritual healing.

Most of the growing interest in spiritual healing in the last century happened largely outside conventional religious organisations. The National Federation of Spiritual Healers, for example, which was started in 1955 is not linked to any religion. It now has 6,000 members in the UK who work in hospitals, doctors surgeries, healing centres and in their own homes.

Healing has become respectable – just as the founders of the NFSH always hoped it would – and today healing is recognised as a complementary therapy by the NHS. This means that your GP may refer you to a healer and you may ask for a healer to visit you in hospital.

## Aesculapius, the first healer

Apollo had a son called Aesculapius who was the Greek god of medicine. We do not know whether he was a real person or a myth, but temples were built in his name dating back to around 1,000 BC.

People used to sleep in these temples in the hope of being visited by the god and having a healing dream.

According to the myth, Aesculapius was brought up by the centaur Chiron who taught him hunting and medicine. Aesculapius became such a famous healer that he was accused of thwarting the order of nature and in the myth, Zeus struck him dead with a thunderbolt.

The symbol for Aesculapius was the serpent and the staff – the same symbol which is used today by medical organisations such as the British Medical Association and the British Holistic Medical Association.

## What happens when you have a treatment?

Healers vary in their approach. You will probably be asked what the problem is, and invited to sit on a chair or stool, or lie down on a couch. You may be encouraged to relax, and it sometimes helps to close your eyes. The healer will then prepare themselves in some way. This is known as attunement. Each healer does it in their own way and you probably will not be aware of what is happening.

Healers ask for the healing to come through them, and this request may take the form of a short, silent prayer, or they may imagine white healing light coming up from the centre of the earth and down from the heavens above, filling them with healing light. They may ask for permission for the healing to happen from your higher self, the part of you that is in contact with the divine. It is as if the healer is saying hello, asking for the energy contact to be made so that the healing can happen.

The healing itself may consist of a light touch from the healer, or their hands may stay just a few inches away from your body. You may feel the healing as a warm, tingly sensation, it may be cool, or you may feel nothing much at all. You may even find that your symptoms get worse momentarily, before they are dissolved in the healing process. Some people find they are able to release and heal emotions during the healing. Everybody reacts differently and you may react differently at different times.

After the healing part of the session has finished, the healer will silently thank and release the source of the healing and thank you for receiving the healing. It is as if the healer is saying good-bye to the energetic connection that has made the healing possible. Again, you are unlikely to be aware of this happening, although the healer will let you know that the healing is completed. You may be encouraged to rest for a few moments before you open your eyes.

After a healing session you may feel clear and energised, or relaxed and sleepy. The effect is completely unpredictable.

## What is healing suitable for?

Spiritual healing is suitable for literally anything and everything – from the trivial to the terminal. This therapy can relieve many of the diseases and complaints that older people can suffer from. It can be particularly helpful with people who are dying, helping everyone concerned to feel calmer and more at peace with the situation.

### ADVANTAGES OF THIS FORM OF TREATMENT

- Nothing is required from you – you do not have to get undressed, it is totally non-invasive. All you have to do is receive the healing energy.
- Healing works with animals, babies and even seeds, so you don't have to believe that it works, although it does help if you have an open attitude to it.
- You do not even have to go to a healer, you can receive absent or distant healing where the healer sends the healing to you.

### DISADVANTAGES OF THIS FORM OF TREATMENT

- The effects of healing are totally unpredictable – for example, it may not help with the backache you thought needed healing, but the tinnitus you thought you had got used to may vanish instead. Or you may not feel better physically, but you may feel happier and more optimistic in yourself. The effect of the healing depends on what your own healing force feels is most appropriate for you at any particular time.
- It does not satisfy the logical part of ourselves that wants explanations and reasons.

## SELF-TREATMENT

Is this therapy suitable for treating yourself? The answer to this question is 'Yes'. Try the following self-healing meditation which comes from *Moon Over Water* by Jessica Macbeth.

- Sit in a comfortable chair with your back straight and your feet on the ground.
- Start by taking a few deep breaths, allowing yourself to settle into relaxation as you exhale, becoming just as relaxed as is comfortable for you at this time.
- There is an energy centre just below and forward of the base of your spine. Please focus your awareness in that centre. This is the root centre. You may be able to feel or to sense the energy in that centre in some way, perhaps as a tingling, or warmth or some other sensation, or perhaps you won't – it doesn't matter, jut be aware that it is there and focus your attention on that part of your body.
- There is another centre of energy at the crown of your head. Please focus your awareness in that centre. This is the crown centre. You may be able to feel or to sense the energy in that centre in some way, perhaps as tingling or coolness or some other sensation, or perhaps you won't – it doesn't matter, just be aware that it is there and focus your awareness in that part of your body.
- There is a line of light that flows from the crown to the root, from the root to the crown. This line of light flows through the centre of your being. Allow your focus of awareness to flow down the line of light from the crown to the root and up from the root to the crown. You may be able to see or to sense the energy flowing along that line of light. If you are, fine; if you're not, just imagine it.
- There is a centre of balance on the line of light. As you follow the flow of the energy from the root to the crown, the crown to the root, be aware of that centre of balance. Breathe into the centre of balance.
- As you breathe into the centre of the line of light, be aware of the breath energising the centre and of the entire line becoming brighter and stronger.
- Be aware of the line of light flowing from the centre of your being down through the root centre, down through your legs and feet, into the earth, and on down to the centre of the earth.

- Feel the line of light connecting your centre with the heart of the earth.
- Be aware of any confusion and tension and static within you, and allow it to drain down this line of light into the earth. Be aware of the earth taking this energy, cleansing and purifying, transforming and strengthening it, and returning it to you as warm, powerful, loving, nurturing energy.
- Allow yourself to become aware of that nurturing, warm energy of the earth, lifting up through you, lifting and cradling every cell of your being. Be aware of the energy rising through your feet and through your entire being.
- Breathe in again to the centre of the line of light, the centre of your being.
- Follow the line of light from the centre of your being upward, up through your crown, to the centre of the universe. Be aware of it rising to the source of the creative life force.
- Be aware of the energy at the centre of the universe, the vital force of life, the source of wisdom, of creation, of compassion. Allow yourself to feel that powerful, wise, creative and loving energy radiating down the line of light into your being. Allow it to flow down through your crown, through the centre of your being, down through your root centre, and into the earth.
- Be aware of the earth's energy rising through you like a warm fountain.
- Be aware of the energy flowing down through you, like living light illuminating every particle of your being.
- Be aware of the warm energy of the earth in the centre of your being. Be aware of the sparkling energy of the heavens in the centre of your being. Experience these energies combining and radiating through your entire being.

## Reiki healing

Reiki, or the Usui system of natural healing, is a form of spiritual healing which has become very popular in the past few years.

Reiki (pronounced Ray-Key) was founded by Dr Mikao Usui in the late 19th century. It is the result of Dr Usui's seven year search for the key to healing. After studying the scriptures and Buddhism, he learned Sanskrit so that he could read the original Buddhist writings where he discovered the formula, symbols and description of how Buddha healed. But knowledge of healing wasn't enough, he wanted the power to heal. So he climbed one of Japan's sacred mountains and meditated for 21 days.

On the twenty-first day, Dr Usui became aware of a beam of light from the heavens that came shooting towards him and knocked him over. Then he saw bubbles of light with the same symbols that he had discovered while he was studying the key to the healing of Buddha and Jesus. The symbols burned themselves into his memory.

When the trance was over, Dr Usui no longer felt exhausted, stiff, or hungry as he had just moments earlier. When he came down from the mountain, he stubbed his big toe, but when he held it the pain left and the bleeding stopped. The first person who he gave healing to had toothache, the second had arthritis – both were cured. He decided to heal the sick in a beggar camp, but after seven years he began to see those he had helped returning to the beggar camp in the same condition that he had originally found them. Dr Usui realised that he had healed the physical body of symptoms but had not taught appreciation for life or a new way of living. He left the beggar camp and began to teach others who wished to know more. He taught them how to heal themselves and gave them the Principles of Reiki.

At the end of his life, Dr Usui recognised Chujiro Hayashi, a retired Naval officer, as the Master of Reiki and charged him with keeping the essence of his teachings intact. Japanese–American Mrs Hawayo Takata became his successor, and she passed her guardianship of the Reiki tradition onto her granddaughter, Phyllis Furumoto.

Dr Usi made a huge commitment when he went on his search for Reiki and a commitment is still demanded of would-be Reiki healers, which is reflected in the high price of learning Reiki. Dr Usui's first healing was on himself – which is the first stage of Reiki. Although Dr Usui was initiated into the power of Reiki very dramatically, today's Reiki healers don't have to meditate on mountains. Students are initiated by a Master, who passes the energy of the symbols into the student's energy field by using symbolic gestures.

The word 'Reiki' means 'universal life force energy'. It is not surprising therefore that it is very similar to other forms of spiritual healing – although it is more structured. A Reiki session usually takes an hour – the healer's hands are placed in twelve positions in all, four on the head, four on the front and four on the back and each position is maintained for five minutes.

## Resources

*Spiritual Healing – A Patient's Guide*, by Eileen Inge Herzberg. C.W. Daniel, 1998.

*Moon Over Water*, by Jessica Macbeth. Gateway, 1990. A useful guide to meditation with lots of different techniques and helpful advice. Includes self-healing exercises.

# Homeopathy

Homeopathy is the treatment of like with like – it means 'similar suffering' in Greek. The theory behind homeopathy is that what causes an ailment can also cure it. Homeopathy uses diluted doses of plants, minerals and animal products such as bee stings.

## History of homeopathy

Although the principle that like cures like has been around at least since the time of Hippocrates, the idea of diluting medicine and experimenting with it on healthy volunteers is comparatively recent. It was invented in the 18th century by the German doctor, Samuel Hahneman (1755–1843). Hahneman spent part of his childhood being educated at home and his parents encouraged him to ask questions and nurtured his inquisitive mind, so perhaps it is not surprising that he became a rebel, questioning medical authority and accepted thinking. He only practised orthodox medicine for nine years before he decided that he couldn't bear to use the cruel methods of blood letting, leeches, or the poisonous, lead-based medicines any longer.

Hahneman 'retired' to live a simple life studying chemistry, writing and translating. The translating work was essential to support his family, but it also gave him food for thought. The key translation was *A Treatise on Materia Medica* by Dr William Cullen, a Scottish physician, teacher, and chemist. The part of the book that aroused Hahneman's curiosity was the 20 pages on Peruvian bark (the source of quinine).

Cullen thought Peruvian bark was successful in treating malaria because it tasted so bitter. But this explanation didn't satisfy Hahneman, so he tried some himself as an experiment. He found that: 'Peruvian Bark, which is used as a remedy for intermittent fever, acts, because it can produce symptoms similar to those of intermittent fever in healthy people'.

The idea that the same medicines that can cure people of disease can actually create these same symptoms in healthy people was an exciting and revolutionary discovery. Hahneman and his colleagues began to experiment on themselves by taking different remedies and keeping detailed records of the symptoms they produced. Hahneman called these experiments 'provings' and it was these provings which formed the foundation for homeopathy. These provings produced symptoms which were similar to illnesses which conventional medical science couldn't help. The medicines used in these provings were then tried on 'incurables' who became healthy again after taking the remedies which were prescribed on the basis of like curing like.

Many of the remedies were made from poisonous substances, but Hahneman found that if he diluted the substance it became harmless, and if he shook it with every dilution, it kept its healing qualities. It didn't just stay the same, the effects actually become more profound every time the substance is diluted and shaken. This process is known as potentisation (see the box on 'How homeopathic remedies are made' overleaf).

In 1810, the first edition of Hahneman's book *The Organon of the Rational Art of Healing* was published. It was the result of 20 years of experimentation and observation, and it set out the principles of homeopathy and described his experiments with different strengths of remedies.

When Hahneman was 80, his wife had died and he was being looked after by his daughters, and he was coming to the end of his life. But he met and fell in love with a 35-year-old Parisian called Melanie. This rejuvenated him, and he went to live in Paris with her. Homeopathy started to take off as the royal and the rich come to be treated by Hahneman and Melanie. When Hahneman died at the age of 88, he was buried in Paris, but there are also monuments to him in Washington DC and other parts of the world.

## How homeopathic remedies are made

First the substance is dissolved in alcohol; this is known as 'the mother tincture'. The mother tincture is mixed with 99 parts of alcohol and then vigorously shaken. This is known as 'the centesimal potency'. Healthfood shops, Boots and other chemists usually stock homeopathic remedies at the 6c potency. The c refers to the centesimal potency and this means that the mother tincture is diluted with 99 parts of alcohol, one part is taken away, diluted 99 times and shaken, and the whole process repeated six times. The alcohol is then poured onto sugar tablets.

Homeopathic remedies can be diluted and shaken many times to make different strength potencies. The remedies may be 6c, 30c, or 200c. Higher potencies are diluted as much as a thousand times, and are known as 1M, 10M or even 50M. ('M' is the Roman numeral for thousand). The higher the potency, the more often it is shaken (or successed) and the more potent the remedy. These higher potencies are used by professional homeopaths.

## *What happens when you have a consultation?*

Much of what happens when you have homeopathic treatment depends on the style of the homeopaths. Some may let you just talk and ask very few questions, others will ask a lot of questions. But whatever the style, all homeopaths are trying to do the same thing. They are all trying to understand you and your symptoms so that they can find the best homeopathic remedy for you.

As they are trying to get to the root cause of your problems, they will be interested in your medical history – what illnesses, drugs and treatments you've had. The homeopath will also want to know what triggered your illness – if for example, you've never been well since you had the flu or a flu jab, or whether your health has deteriorated since your spouse died.

The kind of information they are looking for can be quite surprising. For example:

- What position do you sleep in (on your left side, right side, tummy or back)?
- When are your symptoms at their worst?
- What makes you feel better?
- What makes you feel worse?
- What is your favourite food?
- What foods do you dislike?
- How do you react to hot weather/cold weather?
- Are you sociable or reclusive?
- What are you frightened of?

The homeopath is interested in all your bodily functions:

- How you breathe
- How you deal with exertion
- How you deal with food – from your appetite, or lack of it, to how you eliminate it
- Your circulation – for example, whether your hands and feet are particularly sensitive to cold.

Even if you find it difficult to talk about yourself, the fact that you find it difficult will help the homeopath find the most appropriate remedy for you. As there are thousands of different remedies to choose from, finding the right remedy can be a difficult and time-consuming process.

The homeopath may look through various books and may even use a computer to help make the decision about the best remedy for you. The first consultation will last an hour or more. The homeopath may be able to choose the most appropriate remedy straightaway or may need time to think about it. If you aren't given a homeopathic remedy at the end of the consultation it will normally be sent to you within a few days.

The remedy itself is usually in tablet form, but it may also be granules or powders which dissolve in your mouth or you may be given a liquid remedy.

## What happens next?

Once you have taken the remedy you may notice some changes. You may experience:

- A dramatic feeling of euphoria or well-being.
- A gradual sense of feeling happier in yourself.
- A dramatic improvement in your symptoms.
- A gradual improvement in your symptoms.

Alternatively, you may feel dramatically worse, or slightly worse.

Sometimes the healing that follows the right homeopathic remedy is almost miraculous and there is an extraordinary shift from illness to health. This is particularly common when homeopathy is used for babies and children. However, the older you are, the more slowly and gently the remedy is likely to work. Although you may feel much, much better straight away, it is more likely to be a gradual process. For example, if you suffer from headaches, you may notice that they reduce in intensity and frequency over a period of time.

Sometimes the healing process which follows homeopathic treatment is so subtle that you may not even be aware that anything has happened. It may only be when your homeopath asks about your original symptoms that you realise how much better you feel!

Homeopaths have noticed that the way people get better follows particular patterns – which are exactly the same as the patterns which naturopaths recognise. For example, people get better in the reverse order to the way they became ill (see page 67, the section on 'What naturopaths expect from their treatment').

Homeopathic remedies are sensitive and can be easily spoiled. You should not consume coffee or other drinks containing caffeine while you are undergoing homeopathic treatment. Don't put anything else in your mouth for 10–20 minutes before taking the remedy and 10–20 minutes afterwards. This means:

- No food
- No drink
- No toothpaste
- No smoking.

Homeopathic remedies should be stored in a cool dark place away from anything with a strong smell. If you travel, do not let the remedies go through the x-ray baggage check.

## What is homeopathy suitable for?

Because homeopathy is an energy medicine which works with your own healing energy it can be used to help any complaint you may be suffering from. However, like other forms of natural medicine it cannot reverse physical damage – so for example, if you have osteoarthritis, homeopathy cannot reverse the wear and tear that has already affected the joint. But what it can do is ease the pain, bring more freedom of movement and slow the progress of the disease.

Homeopathy is particularly useful in situations where:

- No one knows what is wrong with you and tests show you are normal, even though you feel unwell.
- When you are suffering from a long term disease where conventional medicine can't help.
- You cannot take drugs.
- You keep getting acute diseases – for example, if you keep getting colds or flu.

### ADVANTAGES OF HOMEOPATHY

- Homeopathic remedies cannot cause side-effects and you cannot become addicted to them.
- Very little is demanded of you in the way of changing your diet or lifestyle (although you may be asked to give up coffee).
- The healing process is gentle and deep and you may notice an improvement quite quickly.

### DISADVANTAGES OF HOMEOPATHY

- Homeopathic treatment is only effective if the homeopath finds the most appropriate remedies – and it can take time and persistence before the right remedies are found.

- Coffee, peppermint, preparations containing menthol, eucalyptus and camphor can all be used as antidotes to homeopathic remedies. Some homeopathic remedies are more likely than others to be prevented from working by caffeine.
- Homeopathic remedies may also be rendered ineffective by dental treatment, conventional drugs or operations.
- Some homeopaths find it hard to find the best remedy for you if you are also taking other forms of medicines.

**SELF-TREATMENT**

Is homeopathy a suitable therapy to use for treating yourself? It is best to visit a professional homeopath for most problems, but there are some homeopathic remedies which it is useful to have in the first aid box:

- **Arnica**     For bruises
- **Calendula**  For cuts, grazes
- **Hypericum**  For puncture wounds.

## Resources

*Healing with Homeopathy*, by David Chappell and David Andrews. Gill & Macmillan, 1996.

*Homeopathy for the Soul*, by Cassandra Lorius. Thorsons, 2001.

# Flower remedies

Flower remedies use the energy of flowers for healing.

## History

Flower remedies can be traced back to the 16th century Swiss doctor and philosopher known as Paracelsus who used dew collected from flowers to cure his patients emotional problems. The idea was rediscovered by homeopath and bacteriologist Dr Edward Bach (1880–1936). While he was recovering from a severe illness, Bach found that he could intuitively understand the healing properties of particular plants.

In 1930, Bach gave up his Harley Street practice and moved to Wales to focus on his work with plants. He believed the flower dew contained the healing properties of the plant and collected this dew for his patients. As more and more people got to hear about Bach's flower remedies, the doctor could not keep up with the demand. He experimented and found that floating freshly picked flowers on clear spring water in sunlight had the same effect. The water is then strained and preserved in alcohol (usually brandy). Making the remedies in this way enabled him to make them in bigger quantities and sell them to a wider public. Today, Bach flower remedies are still made in the same way and widely available in chemists and health-food shops – as well as over the Internet.

Bach believed that physical health was affected by our emotional health and the remedies focus on our emotions. There are 38 Bach Flower remedies which are all concerned with emotional states. For example:

**Olive**        Exhaustion, feeling drained of energy by long-standing problems.
**Gorse**        Feelings of hopelessness, pessimism, defeatism.
**Mimulus**      Fear of known things, shyness, timidity.
**Honeysuckle**  Living in the past, nostalgia, homesickness.

Since the 1980s, many new flower essences have emerged which have been taken from plants growing all over the world including Scotland, California, the Himalayas, Australia, the Amazon and Alaska. Some of these new remedies act on the physical level as well as on the emotions. For example: Australian flower essences include peach flowered tea tree, which helps regulate blood sugar levels as well as fear of ageing.

## What happens when you have a treatment?

The flower remedies are often used in combination with other therapies such as healing and counselling so the methods of treatment may vary.

1  The therapist will try to find out what the underlying problem is. To do this they may ask you some questions, or they may use a pendulum to dowse the appropriate remedy (see the box overleaf).

2 Having decided on the most appropriate remedy or remedies, the therapist will put a few drops in a small bottle and top it up with pure spring water (some people use brandy because the alcohol acts as a preservative).

3 You will be given instructions on how often to take the remedy – usually four drops of the diluted remedy, four times a day. Dr Bach suggested that you imagine that the remedy is filling you with healing light as you take the remedy.

Stop taking the remedy when you feel you no longer need it, and start taking it again if your symptoms come back.

## Dowsing

Dowsing is usually associated with finding underground water or minerals using a dowsing rod or pendulum (a weight on a thread). Bach flower remedy therapists sometimes dowse for the right remedy by using a pendulum to tap into their intuitive knowledge. The therapist will either hold it over the remedies themselves or they may use a special circular chart (published by the Bach Centre) which describes all the remedies.

## What are flower remedies suitable for?

The flower remedies are wonderful for any kind of emotional problem or trauma. They can be particularly helpful during bereavement, or any time of great change.

### ADVANTAGES OF THIS FORM OF TREATMENT

• Flower remedies are gentle and subtle and unlikely to push you into a healing reaction.

### DISADVANTAGES OF THIS FORM OF TREATMENT

• The flower remedies can be so subtle, you may not think that they are having any kind of effect.
• Flower remedies are only effective if the most appropriate one has been chosen.

- If you do not wish to use alcohol, mention this to your practitioner so that they can use water, rather than brandy to make up your remedy.

### Self-treatment

Flower remedies are very suitable for self-treatment, Dr Bach was particularly concerned that they should be simple enough for anyone to use. However, it can be quite difficult to be objective enough about yourself to choose the best remedy.

## Rescue remedy

This is essential for any first aid kit and useful to keep in your handbag (particularly if you are going to a funeral). It is good for shock, accidents and sudden trauma or illness. It also comes in cream form for cuts, grazes, burns and bites.

Rescue remedy is a combination of five remedies:

- **Cherry plum**      For tension, fear, uncontrolled or irrational thoughts
- **Clematis**      For inattention, dreaminess, absent-mindedness, escapism
- **Impatients**      For impatience, irritability
- **Rock rose**      For sudden alarm, fear or panic
- **Star of Bethlehem** For all the effects of serious news, shocks etc.

# 7

# Talking Therapies

## Introduction

The talking therapies help us to focus on our thoughts and emotions. Our thoughts and emotions react to trauma, stress and accidents, in a very similar way to our bodies. We become tense, fearful and think about ways of avoiding getting hurt again.

Whether it is the pain of a car crash or the end of a relationship, the talking therapies can help us to cope with the different layers of our pain. It is not just the injuries themselves that can carry on hurting, our reactions can also make things worse. For example, we can get into the habit of avoiding using an injured limb, and damaging the healthy one in the process. We can also hurt ourselves by avoiding love because it has hurt us in the past.

The talking therapies can help us to release some of the mental and emotional damage that we have experienced in the course of our lives – and help us to stay young at heart.

## *Healing the present*

Only a small proportion of our current aches and pains, be they physical or emotional, belong in the present. The talking therapies can help you to sort out how much of your pain is real and current, how much is left over from the past, and how much involves fretting about the future. If you are recently bereaved for example, the actual bereavement process is very real and current — but that is only part of the picture. Bereavement is also concerned with letting go of the past, and facing up to fears about the future. All the different aspects of the bereavement process are real – and the talking therapies can help you to deal with them.

## Healing the past

The talking therapies can help you to put the past into perspective. Just because something difficult or unpleasant happened in your childhood or in your more recent past, doesn't mean to say that it has to carry on hurting you. The talking therapies can help to reach the point of acceptance, where you have released the pain of the past and can treasure the lessons it has taught you.

## Healing the future

Sometimes what is really hurting us is a fear of the future. The pain is not too bad now, but how will we cope if it gets worse? We may be expecting to be lonely, to have an operation or even to die. The talking therapies can help us to put our fears and anxieties about the future into perspective. They can give us the means to distinguish between what is real and what is simply free-floating anxiety.

Talking therapies can help us to decide what we need to do to avoid our worst fears being realised – or help us to come to terms with the inevitable.

## What's next?

The talking therapies can also help you decide what you want to do with the rest of your life. The second half of life is a challenge to do all the things that you didn't have time for when you were younger. If you have spent a lot of time looking after your family or helping others, now is the time to focus on yourself. This may be the time in your life when you ask such questions as, 'Who am I?' 'What is life about?' When we are young, we hope that we'll know the answer to these questions 'when we get older'. No wonder we sometimes feel depressed when the calendar tells us we are older, yet we find ourselves no wiser!

Provided you are reasonably healthy, there is less that you have to do and more choice in what you can do. Now is the time when you can really do what you want to do because:

- The children have left home.
- There is an increased possibility of living alone because of divorce, and the death of a partner becomes more likely.
- You are likely to be retired or otherwise out of the world of work.

But finding out what you really want to do can be difficult, particularly if your sense of identity has been tied up with looking after your partner, the family and/or your career. It is not always easy to make choices if you've spent 50 years or more doing what's been demanded of you.

No one can tell us how to live this part of our lives. The challenge is to find out what we want to do, what excites and interests us. If we are not used to exploring these questions, some of the talking therapies can be helpful.

## *Healing relationships*

The talking therapies focus on healing many different types of relationship, for example:

- Our relationship with ourselves
- Our relationship with our partners
- Our relationship with our family
- Our relationships with what we do with our lives.

This means that the quality of the relationship between you and your therapist is very important. If you have had problems relating to yourself and others then the talking therapies can give you a new experience of what relationships can be about. This is why it is so important for the talking therapists to have therapy themselves.

## *Death and dying*

At some point, we will all die and, in a sense, what we are all doing is preparing for death. And the things we need to do, in order to die well, are the same as those we need to do in order to live well. These may be practical things such as writing a will, emotional things such as forgiving, or simply allowing ourselves to really enjoy the little things in life such as the smell of a rose. Again, it is the talking therapies that can help us to overcome the obstacles to living life to the full.

## Mind–body, body–mind

Just as the physical therapies also have an effect on our emotions, so our emotions can have an effect on our physical bodies. In fact there is a whole new science with the grand title of 'psychoneuroimmunology' which focuses on this mind/body communication.

Russian physiologist Ivan Pavlov (1849–1936) found that if he rang a bell and then offered meat to a dog several times, the dog would soon respond to the bell as if it were meat – by salivating and licking – even when there was no food. Dr Robert Ader came up with an even more impressive finding. He found that laboratory rats who were given saccharine and an immuno-suppressant drug suffered severe depressions of their immune functions when they were later fed saccharine alone. It appears that the rats got so used to the drug response associated with the saccharine that they continued to react as if they had been given the drug itself. We are at least as intelligent as dogs and rats and these experiments suggest that there are strong links between the way we think and feel and what happens in our bodies.

In the early 1980s, Dr Candace Pert discovered 'messenger chemicals' – neuropeptides – which she called 'the molecules of emotion'. These emotional molecules allow the brain and body to communicate with each other, so that what we think of as our brain is really in every cell of our bodies. There is a continuous link between what we think and what we feel. For example, if you think of eating a lemon, your mouth may pucker up. Compare this to the way your mouth will feel if you think about eating chocolate.

There are several ways in which the talking therapies can affect our bodies. Hypnosis, for example, can have very tangible results, particular in areas such as pain relief, anaesthesia or relaxation. More indirect effects can be seen with counselling and psychotherapy. You may find that one of these talking therapies helps you to understand a long-standing problem in your life and, in the process, a physical pain may disappear.

Just as the talking therapies can have an effect on our physical health, so physical problems can affect us mentally and emotionally. The talking therapists should complement (not replace) more physical approaches.

If you feel that you are on an emotional roller coaster, unusually depressed or anxious, then there may be physical reasons behind this. For example, you may have:

- Diabetes
- Thyroid problems
- Hormone changes (associated with menopause or withdrawal from hormone replacement therapy, for example)
- The after-effects of a heart attack.

It is a good idea to make sure that any physical problems are diagnosed and treated, even if you also go to a therapist as well.

If you are taking medicines which have been prescribed by your doctor, make sure that they are actually making your symptoms better – not worse. For example, *The Health of Adult Britain* 1841–1994 edited by John Charlton and Mike Murphy for the Office for National Statistics quotes various studies which show that:

- 16 per cent of psychiatric hospital admissions amongst older people were caused directly by the ill-effects of drugs, such as sleeping pills and tranquillisers, which affect the mind.
- At least 20 per cent of admissions were precipitated by the adverse effects of mind-altering drugs.
- 21 per cent of the 70–79 age group suffered from adverse drug reactions.

Recreational drugs can also have emotional side-effects. Under the heading 'drugs', we can include almost anything that can make you 'high' – whether it be marijuana, alcohol, coffee or a bar of chocolate. That wonderful mellow feeling you get when you eat chocolate can be followed by a sudden fall in blood sugar when it burns itself out, and low blood sugar can make you feel very tearful and emotional.

Low blood sugar (hypoglycaemia) is very difficult for a GP to diagnose, unless you happen to have a hypoglycaemic attack while you are at the doctor's surgery. The best way of dealing with this is to eat little and often – and avoid sugar. In fact, not eating properly can have a dramatic effect on your emotions. If you are hooked on sugar you may need help from a nutritional therapist who will help you find out whether there is a nutritional problem behind the craving.

You may have good reason to feel depressed, anxious or fearful, particularly if you are in pain, suffering from a long-standing or terminal illness. But it is in exactly these sorts of situations that the talking therapies may be particularly useful. They can help you to find your own inner strengths, and these will help you to cope.

The exciting thing about the talking therapies is that they can enrich your life by helping you to understand who you are, and what you want from life. At their best, these therapies can help you to touch something that is much greater than you are, helping you to come to terms with both living and dying.

## Mental health problems and the talking therapies

According to the mental health charity MIND, one in four of us every year will experience some form of mental health problem ranging from a mild panic attack to a serious mental illness. According to a survey of published research carried out by the Mental Health Foundation (*The Fundamental Facts* by Lisa Bird, 1999), an estimated 15 per cent of people over 65 have depression and an estimated 5 per cent have severe depression. Older people are less likely to be diagnosed as having depression. In a sample of older patients with depression, GPs only recognised 51 per cent as having depression. This group of patients doesn't necessarily receive the right treatment either – the same publication found that 90 per cent of older people who had depression were not treated with the appropriate drugs. People who are depressed often say they feel confused and have difficulty in thinking and remembering things. It's important to find out whether these difficulties are due to depression or to the development of dementia – for example in Alzheimer's disease or after a stroke.

Whether or not the talking therapies can be used in situations where a person is seriously mentally ill (with schizophrenia for example), depends largely on whether the person has support and feels strong enough to face up to and remember difficult situations from the past and, whether they are able to focus and relate to a therapist.

Another Mental Health Foundation survey (*Knowing our Own Minds*, 1997), found that 70 per cent of respondents had experience of talking treatments, and 88 per cent of those who had tried talking therapies found them 'helpful' or 'helpful at times'.

## Resources

*Psychoneuroimmunology* (2nd edition), edited by R. Ader, D. Fellen and N. Cohen. Academic Press, 1990

*The Fundamental Facts*, Lisa Bird for The Mental Health Foundation, 2000. This report contains summaries of research about depression and older people, as well as other mental health issues.

*All about Depression* by Dr Jo Borrill. A free leaflet published by The Mental Health Foundation

*Living with Cancer* by Dr Rosy Daniel. Robinson, 2000.

# Counselling

Counselling is a talking and listening therapy, which helps people who want to deal with a crisis and change their lives and relationships. It can also be an opportunity for them to explore their feelings.

## History of counselling

Since counselling is basically a process of talking and being heard, it is probably as old as language itself. Traditionally, counselling was part of the spiritual life of the community where it was the task of the healer or priest to care for the emotional and spiritual needs of the people. As church attendance fell, more people turned to doctors for help. But with only a few minutes to spend with each patient, the situation was far from ideal, so perhaps it is not surprising that counselling was one of the first complementary therapies to be welcomed into GPs surgeries.

## Counselling in general practice

In the late 1990s, some 40 per cent of fund-holding GP surgeries in England and Wales employed a counsellor.

Around two million counselling treatments were carried out each year.

(Source: *The Fundamental Facts*, by Lisa Bird, published by the Mental Health Foundation, 1999)

### What happens when you have a counselling session?

In the first session, the counsellor will explain what counselling is and together you will explore whether it can help you. You will discuss the problems that you would like to deal with and what you want to achieve. The counsellor will also give you the opportunity to ask them any questions you may have about the nature of counselling, and how it may help you. You will also come to an agreement about what you want to achieve, how often you will meet, and for how long.

After the first session, 'treatment' will consist broadly of:

- You talking
- The counsellor listening
- The counsellor summarising what they have heard you say
- The counsellor making suggestions and/or giving you feedback
- You deciding what to do with what you have said and heard.

The counselling session gives you an opportunity to talk about yourself – and hear yourself speak. The counsellor's role is to help you with this process, by listening to you very carefully, giving you feedback and suggesting techniques which will help.

A good counsellor will make you feel at ease and free to talk, you should feel you can trust them so you can reveal your feelings and thoughts, knowing that what you say will be heard in a non-judgmental, non-critical way, and that you will not be pushed into talking about things you are not ready to deal with. Anything you say will be treated in confidence which means it will not be repeated to anyone else.

The counsellor may sum up and give you feedback about what you have talked about, and point out any recurring patterns. If you are in the process of trying to make a decision, the counsellor may help you summarise the case for and against the various options, but any decision is yours and they will not try to push you in one direction or another.

Counselling sessions last for 50 minutes to an hour and it is usually helpful to go once a week. At the end of a good counselling session you may gain some insight into yourself or the situation you find yourself in. You may also feel lighter and realise the truth in the saying 'a problem shared is a problem halved'.

## What is counselling suitable for?

If you are depressed or anxious, counselling can give you valuable insights into what is really happening in your life, and how to cope with it. For example, depression is often related to feelings of anger which have not been expressed. Counselling can often help people to find useful ways of expressing their anger, so other people are not hurt.

Counselling can be helpful if you feel you have no one to turn to, and you cannot cope with life.

If you are having problems with friends or relatives, or if you are considering changes in your life (such as moving out of your house) counselling can give you an independent perspective. It can also help terminally ill people and their relatives to come to terms with death and dying. Indeed, it can help with any form of bereavement:

- The loss of a loved one
- The loss of a job
- Loss of status
- Being 'at a loss' because the children have left home
- Feelings of loss and violation after a robbery or assault
- Loss of freedom (caused by your own illness or that of a loved one).

Counselling can also help if you are having to cope with any unusual stresses in your life – for example, if you are suffering from a severe illness yourself, or if you are nursing a partner who is terminally ill. Counselling can also:

- Boost self confidence
- Clarify your situation
- Help you gain insight into your motives and needs
- Help you assess past actions
- Help you work out priorities for the future
- Help you assess your progress.

## ADVANTAGES OF THIS FORM OF TREATMENT

- Counselling can help you understand yourself and your life. It helps you feel more in charge.
- It can save your friendships! It is good to talk with friends, in fact if you have enough really good friends who will listen to you, you may find that you don't actually need counselling. But there are times when you need to talk about the same subject over and over and over again to get it out of your system, and a trained counsellor may be able to shorten this process and take some of the load off your friends.
- As counsellors do not know you socially, they don't know how you normally behave which leaves you free to explore new options, new ways of seeing yourself and the way you live your life.
- Unlike friends, counsellors are trained to listen to you in a way that helps you find your own solutions. This means that counsellors will not tell you how you should behave or what you should do.

## DISADVANTAGES OF THIS FORM OF TREATMENT

- This is not a 'get well quick' method – although it can occasionally produce remarkably swift results.
- It does not give you answers on a plate (or in a tablet). If it is going to work, it is because you have made it work.
- You need to feel ready, willing and able to talk and change, and this may be quite difficult, particularly if you are depressed (see the box on Depression).

It can be tempting to talk to your counsellor rather than your nearest and dearest – but this can put a huge strain on your relationships.

It is important to communicate if you want to have good relationships, so if you feel that your problems may stem from your relationship with your partner or your family, it may be a good idea to have couple or family counselling rather than working on a one to one basis.

Counselling may not be necessary if your emotional problems are rooted in a physical problem, so it is important to have a physical check up and have treatment for anything that may be wrong with you physically. For example, no amount of counselling is going to help if you have a thyroid problem. On the other hand, if your depression or anxiety has been caused by the aftermath of a heart attack, counselling can help you understand your feelings which is an important part of your recovery process as your emotional heart will need healing just as much as your physical heart.

Counselling may result in change and disruption in your life. Sometimes what appears to be an emotional problem can be a simple question of logistics and the answer might be to move home. For example, feelings of loneliness could be resolved by moving closer to the rest of the family, feelings of not being able to cope and not having enough money may be resolved by moving to a smaller house.

## SELF-TREATMENT

Counselling requires someone to listen to you – talking to yourself isn't very useful! However, the counsellor may suggest things you can do to help yourself inbetween sessions. For example, your therapist may suggest you keep a diary, or that you become more consciously aware of particular kinds of behaviour.

## Are you depressed?

When you are in the middle of a depression, it is sometimes hard to realise that something is wrong, particularly if it continues for a long time. It can feel as if those dark feelings have become 'normal'. Signals to watch out for include:

- Early waking or problems getting to sleep
- Eating too much or too little
- Loss of libido (sexual appetite)
- Using more tobacco, alcohol or other drugs than usual
- Having less energy and doing less
- Difficulty in concentrating or making decisions.

Other signals to watch out for include:

- Feelings of numbness, emptiness and despondency
- An unusual level of irritability or impatience
- Inability to enjoy normally pleasurable activities
- Self-destructive or suicidal thoughts or actions
- Bleak, pessimistic views of the future
- Finding it difficult or impossible to ask for help or support.

## Different types of counselling

Counsellors may be trained in many different types of counselling and it is important that you feel comfortable both with your counsellor and with their style of approach. Your counsellor may be trained in some of the techniques mentioned in the Psychotherapy section which starts on page 169.

Common forms of counselling include integrative counselling, person-centred counselling and cognitive behavioural therapy.

### PERSON-CENTRED COUNSELLING

As the name suggests, this form of counselling is centred around the person and will follow whatever you, the client wants to do. This emphasis on the client was developed by the American Carl Rogers who wanted to encourage self-reliance and self responsibility. It is up to you, the client, to say whether you just want to talk, or whether you want your counsellor to give a great deal of help and tell you what to do. You are in charge of what happens in the session.

## INTEGRATIVE COUNSELLING

The integrative approach means that the therapist has trained in several different approaches to counselling and will use whichever techniques are most appropriate, depending on what you need. 'Integrative' also implies making 'whole', which is how you should feel after receiving counselling.

## COGNITIVE THERAPY

This form of counselling is particularly suitable if you like to take a logical, problem-solving approach to life. It is based on the idea that it is the thoughts we have, rather than external events, which create our moods and so we can change the way we feel and behave by changing the way we think about things.

## BEHAVIOURAL THERAPY

This is another logically-based form of therapy. It is based on the idea that we can change negative thoughts and behaviour by learning 'good' ways of thinking, feeling and behaving. It includes some things that you can do to help yourself, such as recording an activity schedule, as described in the box.

## Activity schedules: an hour by hour record of what you do

Rate each activity between 0 and 10 for pleasure and call that P for pleasure. Rate each activity for achievement and call it M for merit (or A for achievement if you prefer). It is important to do this at the time it is actually happening, not with hindsight. Even sitting in a chair or lying in bed is doing something.

The next step is to plan ahead so that you feel that you are taking control of your life again.

List the things that you have been putting off – prioritise them, break them down into small tasks, identify negative thoughts about doing the task and write them down. Focus on what you have achieved.

### ASTROLOGICAL COUNSELLING

Astrological counselling uses the birth chart as a guide to help the counsellor and the client to understand themselves and the situations they find themselves in. It can be helpful in uncovering hidden aspects of the personality so that these can be recognised and brought into conscious awareness.

### CO-COUNSELLING

In co-counselling, you take turns as counsellor and client. For example, you may decide that, for the first half hour, you will be the client and your co-counselling partner will be the counsellor. During that half hour you will do most of the talking, although your partner may give you suggestions about what to do to help you gain more insight into what you are talking about. After the half hour is up, you change roles and you become the counsellor and your partner becomes the client for half an hour.

Co-counsellors are trained to make appropriate suggestions and to listen attentively. Co-counselling was introduced into England in the 1970s and is sometimes called 're-evaluation counselling'.

## The difference between counselling and psychotherapy

Counselling is concentrated on an agreed length of time – this can be anything from a few weeks to a few months. Psychotherapy is much more open ended and can take several years.

Counselling tends to focus on the conscious mind and the emotions. Psychotherapy is also concerned with other levels of consciousness. Long term psychotherapy will often look to the past and relate it to the present, counselling may help you to look forward and plan ways of making changes.

## Resources

*Bereavement and Grief: supporting older people through loss*, by Steve Scrutton. Co-published by Edward Arnold and Age Concern, 1995.

*Counselling and Older People: An introductory guide*, edited by Verena Tschudin. Published by Age Concern Books, 1999.

*First Steps in Counselling*, by Pete Sanders. A students' companion to basic introductory courses. Published by PCCS Books, 1998.

*Someone to Talk to Directory*. Published on the Internet by the Mental Health Foundation, this directory lists many kinds of counselling services including bereavement, depression, divorce, marriage guidance, sexual problems, stress problems, addiction, family problems and a range of medical disorders.

### Relate

Formerly known as the Marriage Guidance Council, Relate specialises in relationship problems. There are many regional branches and you will find contact details in your local telephone book.

# Psychotherapy

Literally, the therapy of the mind, psychotherapy uses a wide range of techniques to change mood, behaviour, health and consciousness so that life is more satisfying and rewarding. It can also be called 'soul healing'. During a psychotherapy session you may be encouraged to look closely at your past, particularly your childhood and your relationships.

## History of psychotherapy

Modern psychotherapists can trace their roots to ancient healer priests and shamans. Their role was partly to interpret messages from the gods and these messages could take the form of dreams, illness, or natural events. They were also healers and to do this work, they used out of the ordinary states of consciousness or trance states and invoked these states in their patients.

Sigmund Freud (1856–1939) found that hypnosis could help his patients remember long-forgotten traumatic events, and when they re-experienced these traumas, they could recover from chronic physical and emotional problems. Freud suggested that abuse, neglect, serious illness, loss or abandonment, could stop children from developing healthy ways of coping with life. Freudian analysis consisted of past traumas and repressed urges being remembered and acknowledged by the patient who experienced a release of pent-up feelings. This catharsis was part of the healing process, but it was also important to experience re-parenting so that new patterns of behaviour could be learned. The patient is encouraged to relate to the psycho-analyst as a parent figure. To facilitate this, patients usually lie on a couch with the therapist sitting out of sight behind them.

Carl Gustav Jung (1875–1961) was a friend and colleague of Freud, and they were both interested in the revolutionary idea that man has an unconscious mind. But they fell out when Jung developed his own thoughts about the nature of therapy and the interpretation of dreams.

Jung was the first to express the following views:

- There is a wise person within all of us whose voice is heard in dreams and sometimes as an inner voice or prompting.
- Dreams are not the only way that the unconscious makes itself known – waking events and images are also signals from the unconscious.
- Women have an inner male (animus) and men have an inner female (anima).
- The unconscious is divided into the personal unconscious and the collective unconscious.
- Myths and fairy tales are part of the collective consciousness, which they help us to understand.
- Creativity is fuelled by the unconscious – our own, personal unconscious feelings and emotions, as well as collective unconscious material in the shape of archetypal and mythical images.
- One of the roles of therapy is to help us hear this wise part of ourselves and to unleash our creative potential.

Jung wrote 20 books and his ideas hugely influenced the school of psychotherapy known as 'the growth movement'. It has also been called 'the human potential movement' and 'humanistic psychology'. But it is Abraham Maslow (1908–1976) who is widely regarded as the founding father of humanistic psychology. He focused his attention on health, and wanted to know what made people stable, well-motivated and fulfilled. Maslow studied people who were outstandingly successful and those who had had mystical experiences. He developed the idea of a 'hierarchy of needs'. In this he claimed that when people have got to grips with physical, emotional and social challenges, they can move towards self-actualisation, a state of fully understanding and experiencing the self.

At the time Maslow's ideas were evolving, the developed countries had survived a world war and many people had a reasonable standard of living and were looking for something more than just survival. In the 1960s the 'me' generation were smoking marijuana, experimenting with mind altering drugs such as LSD, and protesting against war. They were also exploring Eastern philosophies and starting to practice meditation, trying to answer that important question 'Who am I?' The seeds of the growth movement were planted and a bewildering array of new therapies sprung up. Perhaps it is not surprising that some of these therapies used altered states of consciousness (see the box).

## Altered states of consciousness

An altered state of consciousness can be anything from a light daydream to deep sleep. The therapies that use altered states of consciousness work with trance states, just like the ancient healer priests and healers.

Just as there are different levels of sleep, so there are different levels of trance:

**1 Light trance** — Your eyes are closed and you are deeply relaxed and open to suggestions.

**2 Medium trance** — All your bodily processes slow down and you won't feel much pain, allergic reactions stop and you are responsive to hypnotic suggestions.

| 3 **Deep trance** | A sleepwalking state where your eyes may be open, but you are very responsive to hypnotic suggestion. This is the state where total anaesthesia is possible. |

Although the growth movement started in California, it spread rapidly to Britain, and some of these therapies have taken root and are growing into respected forms of psychotherapy. In fact most psychotherapists call themselves 'eclectic' which means they have trained in many different methods of psychotherapy and can choose whichever form is most appropriate to the circumstances.

Some of the tools which psychotherapists and counsellors use include:

- Dreams
- Drama
- Guided imagery
- Visualisation
- Hypnosis
- Art therapy
- Bodywork
- Writing.

## What happens when you have psychotherapy?

Complementary psychotherapists prefer to call people clients, not patients, and the time spent together is usually called a session rather than a treatment.

Most sessions are client-centred – so what you actually do will depend largely on you. It may be that all you really want to do is talk and be listened to, with no interventions or suggestions from the therapist. On the other hand, you may want the therapist to suggest ways of helping you to get in touch with what is happening underneath the surface. The therapist may do this by encouraging you to focus on:

- The first thing that pops into your head
- Your feelings
- Your breath
- Your body
- Dreams.

## TOOLS PSYCHOTHERAPISTS USE

The therapist may use interventions or suggestions, using different tools to help you contact hidden parts of yourself to give you a deeper insight into yourself and what is happening in your life.

## Gestalt therapy

'Gestalt' is German for 'form' or 'shape'. This therapy was developed by Fritz Perls who became disenchanted with Freudian analysis and interested in a more body–oriented approach. Gestalt therapy uses dream analysis, meditation and bodywork. Gestalt therapists were the first to use cushions to represent different parts of ourselves.

## Bodywork

This describes any therapy which focuses on the body as a means of getting in touch with the emotions.

Wilhelm Reich, the father of bodywork, found that every time we have an emotional shock or trauma, it triggers a series of events where our energy, character and body react in order to protect us from future harm. This is known as 'body armouring'. Reich found that:

- Softening the body armour could release the original trauma.
- Releasing the original trauma could soften the body armour.

This in turn can help us to feel freer, so we can move more easily both physically and emotionally.

Reich's work was developed into bio-energetics by Alexander Lowen who created a series of exercises designed to release body armouring. Reich's theories also played a key role in developing biodynamic massage (see pages 105–107).

## Psychodrama

This technique is based on the idea that acting out your problems and conflicts is much more helpful than just talking about them. It was developed by the Venetian psychiatrist Jacob Moreno, just after World War II. Moreno was inspired by an actress who was unpleasant in her private life when she played sweet and gentle roles, yet became sweet and gentle at home when she was given the stage role of an unpleasant character.

A psychodrama workshop starts with some form of warm up exercise which may be simply talking until it is clear who is 'hot' and ready to work. The drama is then built around them as they describe a scene from their childhood and other members of the group are given roles to play. These parts often resonate with the 'actors', reminding them about incidents from their own childhood. During the course of the drama, the director or therapist may suggest different strategies such as *role reversals* where one person acts as someone else, or *mirroring*, where one person copies another.

Many of the ideas Moreno used in psychodrama are now used by psychotherapists working with individuals as well as for group sessions.

## Art therapy

Painting and drawing can provide important information about what is happening in the unconscious. You are encouraged to paint or draw something – anything that comes into your mind. The therapist will help you to look at the painting in such a way that it can help you to understand what is happening in your life.

## Psychosynthesis

Roberto Assagioli (1888–1974) started this therapy which introduced the ideas of guided imagery and sub-personalities to psychotherapy. Guided imagery is described later in this chapter.

Assagioli was a Freudian psychiatrist who agreed with Jung, that there was more to life than reacting against our parents. Assagioli introduced the idea of a higher, or transpersonal level of consciousness.

Sub-personalities are different parts of ourselves. For example, our unconscious may see a part of ourselves as a princess with servants, and this may be the part of ourselves which is oblivious to such chores as washing up and tidying up.

As the name implies, the idea behind psychosynthesis is to achieve a synthesis, a coming together, of the various parts of ourselves. The connection between the spiritual dimension and the person's 'higher' or 'transpersonal' self is an important part of this therapy. The higher self is a source of wisdom, inspiration, unconditional love, and gives meaning to our lives and is our direct link to the Divine.

## Transpersonal psychology

Psychosynthesis is a form of transpersonal psychology — a term that covers any form of psychology concerned with spiritual or transcendental experiences. It also includes the unconscious parts of ourselves, what Jung calls the 'shadow'. It embraces both the sky and the mountains as well as the dark caves and forests. Transpersonal psychology is concerned with the collective consciousness of symbols, mandalas, myths, fairy tales and archetypes.

In Britain, this form of therapy was pioneered by industrial psychologist Sir Ian Gordon Brown and Barbara Somers, a trained Jungian analyst. Therapists at the Bristol Cancer Help Centre have used transpersonal psychology very successfully to help people understand themselves and their cancer.

## Guided imagery

With this technique you are helped to enter a deeply relaxed trance state, but instead of taking you back to your childhood, you are taken on an inner journey. The journey may be designed in different ways, depending on the purpose of the imagery. It may:

- Help you to gain insight into your current state of mind.
- Help you to gain insight into different aspects of your personality.
- Help you to make contact with a wise part of yourself.
- Help you find your own, wise answers to a problem that is troubling you.
- Help you to make contact with your unconscious motivations.

- Help you to make contact with the Divine.
- Provide a healing experience.

### Visualisation

In visualisation you imagine a situation in the hope of making it come true. This technique has been used at the Bristol Cancer Help Centre with considerable success.

Carl Simonton started using imagery with cancer patients in the 1970s in America. At first Simonton used aggressive images like sharks attacking and killing cancer cells, but he later found that it was more effective to use more positive, relaxing, calming images of cancer cells being healed and carried out of the body.

## *What is psychotherapy suitable for?*

Psychotherapy is helpful if you are moving into a new phase of life, dealing with loss or change in such areas as work, health, home or relationships. It can also be helpful if you are feeling a lack of confidence, depression or anxiety. It can improve the quality of your experience of life and deepen your relationship with yourself and others. It can also enrich your self-awareness and creativity and bring meaning into your life. Because of the connection between mind and body, psychotherapy can also be used to help heal physical problems.

#### ADVANTAGES OF PSYCHOTHERAPY

- It provides you with an opportunity for self discovery and growth.

#### DISADVANTAGES OF PSYCHOTHERAPY

- It relies on you wanting to learn about yourself and grow in some way – if you would prefer to stay as you are, then psychotherapy is not for you.

#### SELF-TREATMENT

Psychotherapy is a journey of self discovery and it is usually helpful to have someone who knows what they are doing to accompany you.

## Resources

*Sun Over Mountain*, by Jessica Macbeth. Gateway, 1981. A useful book if you want to work with guided imagery.

# Hypnotherapy

Literally, the therapy of sleep, from the Greek word 'hypnos' to sleep, hypnosis puts you in an out-of-the-ordinary state of consciousness, somewhere between waking and sleeping, so that you can work with the subconscious parts of your self.

## History of hypnotherapy

Dreams carrying messages from the gods were invoked by ancient healers and shamans using herbs and post-hypnotic suggestion. Altered states of consciousness have been an important part of healing traditions as long ago as the ancient Chinese and Egyptians. Hieroglyphs and pictures show Egyptians using hypnotism in religious ceremonies and medical treatment which may have included using it as an anaesthetic in surgery.

In the late 18th century, a Viennese doctor Franz Anton Mesmer (1733–1815) found that when people went into a trance their symptoms disappeared. He called it 'mesmerism' and tried to explain the healing process as stored cosmic fluid and animal magnetism, but was ridiculed by the European medical profession.

James Braid (1795–1860), a Scottish eye surgeon, was sceptical until he saw Mesmer at work. Braid was so impressed with this 'mesmerism' that he used the technique himself, but he called it 'hypnosis'. Braid found that patients who had been hypnotised suffered from less pain and bleeding, recovered more quickly and were less likely to die after operations. Another Scottish surgeon, James Esdaile (1808–1859) performed 300 major operations and 2,000 minor ones using hypnosis as the only anaesthetic.

But the medical establishment was sceptical about hypnotism, and it was not until 1955 that the British Medical Association approved hypnotherapy as a valid medical treatment. Three years later, the American Medical Association gave its approval.

Because modern anaesthetics are so effective, using hypnosis for anaesthesia has gone out of fashion. However, some dentists use hypnotism was well as traditional anaesthetic to relax patients and help control bleeding and salivation (dribbling).

In 1956 the *British Medical Journal* carried an article about skin diseases and psychological conditions being cured by hypnotherapy. Since then there has been a growing interest in the way the mind affects the body (see pages 155–159, 'Introduction to the talking therapies').

## What happens when you have a treatment?

At first the therapist will talk to you about what you would like to achieve with hypnotherapy – and why. This is an important part of the process, because your own conscious ideas will be reinforced while you are under hypnosis. For example, if you want to be hypnotised to help you give up smoking because you are worried about your health, it may be suggested to you that you don't want to smoke and would prefer to be healthy, breathing in only fresh, unpolluted air.

Hypnosis itself is a simple process of encouraging you to be 'more and more relaxed'. This may be done just by talking to you, perhaps counting backwards, or suggesting that you are feeling heavy, warm, and relaxed. Some hypnotherapists also use a focusing device where you concentrate on their finger, or a pendulum.

Everyone can get into a relaxed state of mind. Research suggests that 90 per cent of the general population can be hypnotised, with 20–30 per cent able to go into a deep trance state where anaesthesia is possible (source: Ernest R. Hilgard, *Hypnotic Sensibility*, Harcourt-Brace, 1965).

Exactly what happens under hypnosis depends on the purpose of the session. For example, you may want to achieve something very specific, such as giving up smoking, or it may be part of a psychotherapy process. You can learn more about yourself and your unconscious by using the hypnotic state to help you remember:

- Incidents from your childhood
- Incidents from past lives (known as 'past life therapy')
- Decisions made when you were very young which affect your current behaviour.

Hypnosis can also be used to plant suggestions in your mind, which will only surface in appropriate situations. This is known as 'post-hypnotic suggestion' and can be used to help people change their habits such as giving up smoking, eating less, and so on. Post-hypnotic suggestion can also help with pain control. For example, before an operation, dentistry or medical procedure, a hypnotherapist may suggest that you will feel more and more relaxed and comfortable in those situations where you would normally expect to experience pain.

When hypnosis is used as an anaesthetic, you are put in a very deep hypnotic trance. This altered state of consciousness is so profound that you will not feel any pain.  For best results:

- You should feel comfortable with your therapist, and trust them.
- The room you work in should be comfortable and free from distraction.
- You need to feel willing to take part in the process.

A hypnotherapy session will usually last from between an hour and 90 minutes and you may need to have a session once a week for six to twelve weeks.

## What is hypnotherapy suitable for?

Hypnotherapy can help a wide variety of problems including:

- Depression
- Multiple personalities
- Anxiety
- Bi-polar disorder (sometimes known as manic depression)
- Problems in concentration
- Impotence
- Anorexia
- Insomnia
- Panic.

- Fear of flying
- Stress and neurosis
- Arthritis
- Heart disease
- Hypertension
- Nervous tension
- Headaches
- Irritable bowel syndrome
- Colitis and asthma.

Hypnotism can help you to remember long-forgotten events in this life, or a past life that has had an effect on your health. For example, people with chest and breathing difficulties may find that these problems relate to a difficult birth where the umbilical cord may have been twisted around their neck. Some people believe that chest and breathing problems can be traced to a past life where they drowned.

# Rebirthing

There are several different ways in which you may remember what happened to you when you were born. Hypnotherapy can be used, but it can also happen spontaneously during some forms of psychotherapy such as bodywork. There is also a group of therapists known as re-birthers who specialise in a breathing technique which can help you to remember and release birth traumas.

During a re-birthing session you will be asked to pay attention to the breath, allowing it to deepen and eventually to become circular, with the emphasis on the in-breath, while the out-breath stays soft and relaxed. The idea behind this special breathing is to give you a deep sense of relaxation, which makes it easier to release emotional tension that is held in the body.

The connected breathing of re-birthing copies newborn babies who naturally breathe in a relaxed way, with no pause between the in breath and the out breath. Re-birthing is based on the idea that when we are in pain or frightened in any way, we automatically hold the breath. This forces carbon dioxide back into the blood stream, thus deadening the pain. Using connected breathing can help you to release the original pain or fear and help you to breath more freely. It can also help you to release chemicals such as anaesthetics that may have been affecting you since birth.

Using the breath allows you to relax so deeply that spontaneous images and feelings come to the surface – this may relate to your birth, or it may relate to something else which had a profound affect on your breath and how you live your life.

# 8
# Food Section

## Introduction

This section is about food and nutrition. What we eat – and how much we eat – makes a huge difference to our health and well-being. In fact, nutrition has had a bigger influence on our health than anything else – including modern medicine, according to medical epidemiologist Thomas McKeown.

Food becomes particularly important as we get older because our digestive system becomes less efficient. According to a report featured in *The Times* in January 2001, more than half of older patients admitted to hospitals are suffering from malnutrition. But this is only part of the story. Books and magazines are full of ideas about what we should and should not be eating, and the vitamins and supplements we need to live long, healthy lives. While there is some research to show that there are a number of simple things that you can do to help yourself stay healthy, so far at least, the elixir of eternal youth has proved elusive.

The Department of Health recommends the eating of at least five pieces of fruit and vegetables a day in order to minimise the risk of heart disease. But as you will see in the following section, there are therapists who go much further than this and use food as medicine. In fact the traditional Chinese medicine approach is that 'pills and potions' should only be used if dietary methods fail.

As far as supplements are concerned, there is good evidence to suggest that vitamins A, C and E, known as anti-oxidants, can help the body to fight free radicals, the body's bullies described in Chapter Two. Also, as we get older, it gets more difficult for us to convert sunlight into vitamin D, so it is also a good idea to have vitamin D supplements in the form of fish liver oil tablets. Vitamin D helps us absorb calcium and phosphorus for bone formation, it also helps our nervous system, heart and blood clotting mechanisms.

Some complementary therapists feel that if your own healing energies are working properly, and you eat a well-balanced diet, then you may not need supplements. Others argue that supplements give the body the nourishment it needs in order to stay healthy. Some go even further and say that many of the complaints we associate with ageing are caused by vitamin and mineral deficiencies. Diets and supplements feature strongly in most of the books that focus on staying young and healthy.

As we get older, getting enough nourishment from our food may become more difficult. Digestion is less efficient. The stomach produces less gastric acid, and the pancreas makes fewer digestive enzymes, so fewer of the nutrients from food can be absorbed. Also the gut tends to slow down, which makes constipation more common, so it is particularly important to eat plenty of fibre.

Gum disease and dental problems can spoil the enjoyment and nourishment we get from food. Chewing is the first stage of digestion, so it is important to have regular dental check-ups and ensure that dentures are fitted properly.

Depression, loneliness or having to live on a low income can affect your eating habits. As you get older, particularly if you live on your own, you may find it hard to bother to cook 'proper' meals. But no one can live on digestive biscuits and tea alone, so the single most important thing you can do to improve your health is to find a way of eating properly. If you are well, you might decide to invite friends over for dinner. This has several benefits: it ensures that you have at least one 'proper' meal – more if you count the leftovers. It is also a sociable thing to do, which may be a difficult leap to make if you are depressed, but it is well worth doing.

If you are not well enough for socialising, there are other ways of getting nourishing meals. These include 'meals on wheels' and visiting a day centre, both of which can be arranged through your local social services department.

## Resources

*The New Ageless Ageing* by Leslie Kenton. Published by Vermilion, 2000.

*Naturopathy* by Stewart Mitchell. Published by Blackwell, 1979.

# Dietary therapy

Dietary therapy is concerned with how the food we eat can make us well.

## History of dietary therapy

'Man lives on one quarter of what he eats. On the other three quarters his doctor lives'. This observation was carved on to an Egyptian pyramid more than 5,000 years ago.

Hippocrates invited us 'to let food be thy medicine, and medicine thy food'.

We say 'eat this, it will do you good' – it is so instinctive that it is not surprising that dietary therapy is an important part of all the major forms of traditional medicine.

## Eat seaweed for a long life

The cell structure of adult whales is practically the same as newborn whales and they tend to die of accidents rather than disease. As discussed in Chapter 2, human cells tend to deteriorate with age.

We do not know exactly why whales have such sturdy cells, but seaweed enthusiasts claim it is because of all the seaweed and algae they eat. Certainly seaweeds such as kelp, kombu, and wakame are rich in minerals – and they don't taste nearly as bad as they sound!

(Source: *Healing with Whole Foods*, by Paul Pitchford. North Atlantic Books, 1996)

## *Traditional Chinese medicine (TCM)*

TCM sees food in terms of energy, using it to help balance our physical and energy bodies. The right diet will depend on what is wrong with us. For example:

**Yin**   Upward, rising energy, will be found in upward, rising foods such as leafy green vegetables.

**Yang**   Downward, grounding energy will be found in vegetables that grow downwards such as carrots and other root vegetables.

As we get older, we have less yin and our yang will also tend to decline, but more slowly. How much yin and yang we need will depend on our own body balance. As we get older we tend to be more sensitive to the cold and have less physical energy, so we need to have warming foods and avoid raw food. However, cooling foods can be helpful if you have an inflammatory problem (such as rheumatoid arthritis).

Apart from the foods which are physically warm because they are served cooked and hot, some foods are warming by their very nature. Examples are high protein foods such as fatty meats or eggs. Fried and spicy foods, and ingredients soaked in wine, are also all warming and raise the heat in the body.

Apart from foods which are physically cool because they are served raw and cold, some foods are naturally cooling. For example, celery, lettuce, watercress, fruit, crab and fish are all cooling and reduce heat in the body.

- **Drying foods** include barley, aduki beans, alfalfa and kidney beans.
- **Moistening foods** include milk, eggs, sardines, asparagus, cucumber, olives, soybean, tofu and spinach.

TCM views food as a way of balancing your energies, so if you want to become more yin, then you should eat plenty of yin foods such as leafy green vegetables, if you want to become more yang, then eat more yang food such as root vegetables.

## Eat young to stay young

Eating young food has a reputation for keeping you young. This does not just mean baby carrots or mangetout, it includes sprouting grains, legumes (beans, peas etc) and seeds. Sprouting is believed to break down the fats, proteins and starches in these foods and makes them easy to digest. It also boosts the nucleic acid contents ten times. Nucleic acid is the vital ingredient in DNA (deoxyribonucleic acid).

To sprout seeds, grains, etc, soak them in water overnight, drain. Leave in a glass or clear plastic container in a dark, warm place for a few days and then put it out in the sun (on a window sill is fine). Rinse and drain twice a day. After a few days they should start sprouting. It is very satisfying to see them grow. You don't need to do many at a time – start off with a teaspoon and see how much (or how little) you need.

## *Ayurvedic medicine*

Ayurvedic medicine also uses food to help balance our physical and energy bodies, and like TCM, Ayurvedic medicine sees food in terms of energy. According to Ayurvedic medicine, what you should be eating depends on the help that your constitution (or dosha) needs to stay in balance – and the time of year. To increase your energy you may be advised to increase spices and meat in your diet. If you want to lower your energy, dairy products may be prescribed.

Ayurvedic medicine describes ageing as a process of increased vata which is a tendency to become drier, thinner, more nervous and restless with less appetite, less sleep and more fear. Because of the drying out process, the likelihood of constipation increases. Bananas and drinking plenty of water can be helpful if you have constipation. Almonds, avocados and coconuts are also recommended.

## *Naturopathy*

Diet is also an important part of naturopathy. Again the emphasis is on bringing you back into balance, so that the kind of diet that is prescribed for you will depend on what your problems are.

The 'back to nature' ideals of the naturopaths are reflected in their approach to diet. Food should be eaten in their natural season, so strawberries for example, should only be eaten in the summer. Naturopaths believe that we should eat the natural, unprocessed foods that our bodies have been learning how to digest over the past five million years. This means eating fresh fruit, vegetables, nuts, eggs, fish and some meat. Cereals and grains should be eaten in their whole, unrefined state – this means eating brown rice and brown bread rather than the white varieties.

Naturopaths believe that when we are well, a large proportion of our diet should be raw, so that none of the nutrients are lost in the cooking process. There are, of course, exceptions. For example, potatoes and grains need to be cooked and not everyone has a digestive system which is strong enough to cope with too much raw food. When you see a naturopath, they will devise a special diet suited to your own individual needs.

### Food tonic

Nettles can be cooked as a green vegetable or used like a herb as a kidney tonic or general pick-me-up. It thickens the hair and enriches the blood. Milarepa, an ancient Tibetan sage, fasted on nettles until his skin turned light green and he developed legendary psychic and physical powers.

Royal jelly and bee pollen also have the reputation of giving you an energy 'buzz'. Royal jelly promotes impressive physical growth, productive ability and longevity for the queen bee. In Chinese medicine it has the reputation for stimulating sexuality and extending life. Some French people take it as a 'cure' for a month or so a year, and Bulgarian researchers have conducted research into its ability to speed regeneration of damaged tissue, lower blood pressure and cholesterol, increase tolerance to stress and improve the immune system.

## *Dietitians*

Dietitians are part of mainstream medicine and their rôle in orthodox medicine has been recognised since the 1930s when the British Dietetic Association was formed. Dietitians are trained to degree level and above and their approach is scientifically based – it is not usually considered to be part of complementary medicine.

Dietitians will talk to you about your normal diet and may ask you to write down everything you eat. This information may be fed into a computer in order to analyse what you eat. The dietitian may then make suggestions on how to adapt your diet according to your needs.

Dietitians specialise in the complaints that can be affected by what you eat. For example, if you have had a heart attack, they will advise you on how to reduce your risk of another heart attack by eating less animal fat and more fruit and vegetables. If you have diabetes, they will help you find ways of controlling your need for insulin by reducing the sugar in your diet, and increasing starches and roughage. Diabetics also have to have a cholesterol-lowering diet because of their increased risk of heart disease.

Nutritional therapists (discussed in more detail in the next section) are complementary medicine practitioners who use special diets and nutritional supplements to help people with a variety of health problems. Apart from these specialist nutritional therapists and traditional medicine practitioners, many other complementary medicine practitioners also offer advice on diet and nutrition.

Dietitians and other nutritionists recommend that you eat a varied diet – we were not made to live on bread alone. Assuming that you do not have special medical problems, dietitians recommend that older people eat:

- One main meal and two snacks.
- Once a day, half a pint of milk in yoghurts etc.

- Twice a day, some form of protein in the form of meat, fish, poultry, eggs, cheese etc.
- At least one serving of cereal such as pasta or breakfast cereal.
- Two to three servings of vegetables.
- One to two servings of fruit (including fruit juice).
- Eight cups of water.

## What happens when you have dietary treatment?

Whatever form of dietary medicine you choose, it will basically consist of several similar steps.

### FINDING OUT WHAT IS WRONG

At this stage the practitioner may ask you about your health – any symptoms you may be suffering from, as well as a brief outline of any problems you may have had in the past. The practitioner will then try and find out which areas are out of balance. Depending on the background of the therapist this may take the form of looking at your tongue, feeling your pulse, asking questions, or taking samples for laboratory analysis.

A dietitian will ask what you normally eat and may analyse this with a computer to see what vitamins, minerals and nutrients are part of your normal diet – and what may be missing. Once the underlying imbalance has been identified, the therapist will suggest a diet that has been tailor-made for you.

You will be asked to come back and discuss your progress at regular intervals.

## Some definitions

| | |
|---|---|
| *Vegetarians* | Vegetarians do not eat meat, but they sometimes eat fish. Vegetarians also eat eggs, cheese, and other dairy products. |
| *Vegans* | Vegans do not eat any animal products, including eggs and dairy products. |

| Wholefood | This refers to unprocessed, unrefined food such as brown rice, wholemeal bread. |
| Organic | This refers to food that has not been grown with the help of pesticides, weedkillers or artificial fertilisers. |
| Macrobiotics | From the Greek words meaning 'large' and 'life', because Japanese writer George Ohsawa, who developed macrobiotics, believed that this approach could make everyone healthy enough to enjoy life to the full. Macrobiotics use the Chinese principles of yin and yang to balance our diet and ourselves. Macrobiotics tend to use a lot of brown rice because it is a well-balanced food, and seaweed because it is rich in minerals and nutrients. |

## What is dietary therapy suitable for?

What we eat is such an important feature in our lives and our health that it is hard to imagine any ailments where diet does not have a part to play. We are what we eat!

Diseases where diet is particularly important include:

- Heart disease
- Diabetes
- Liver and gallbladder problems
- Digestive problems
- Elimination problems ( constipation and diarrhoea)
- Obesity
- Malnutrition.

### ADVANTAGES OF THIS FORM OF TREATMENT

- It is something that you can do for yourself: it helps you to feel in control of what is happening to you.

### DISADVANTAGES OF THIS FORM OF TREATMENT

- It is something that you have to do for yourself: it takes time, effort and commitment.

## SELF-TREATMENT

Is this therapy suitable for treating yourself? The answer to this question is positively, 'Yes'. In fact there are thousands of self-help books that recommend different kinds of diets to help you live longer, look younger and heal yourself of a large range of diseases and complaints. Many of them are based on traditional ideas of eating a largely vegetarian, wholefood diet.

Some of the more popular dietary therapy regimes currently available include the following.

### The Raw Food Diet

This is based on the idea that raw food gives us energy because the vitamins and minerals are not destroyed in the cooking process. It also suggests that because our digestive system is long and narrow, just like those of vegetable-eating animals, it is particularly well equipped to cope with raw vegetables.

Some people find raw vegetables very hard to digest and need them to be cooked to soften the cell walls to help the digestive process. This is particularly important as you get older if you have problems chewing your food.

Recommended reading: *New Raw Energy*, by Leslie Kenton, published by Vermilion, 1994.

### The Bristol Diet

This regime, originally devised by Dr Alec Forbes at the Bristol Cancer Help Centre, was also based on a large proportion of the food being raw. The BCH now recommends that people with cancer have a vegan, low fat diet with 50 per cent cooked food.

Recommended reading: *Healing Foods* by Dr Rosy Daniel, published by Century, 2000

*The Healing Foods Cookbook* by Jane Sen, published by Thorsons, 1996

## 'Eat right for your type'

This diet is based on the idea that your blood group type is a good indicator of what foods you should eat and what illnesses and diseases you are most likely to suffer from if you do not 'eat right'. It was devised by Dr Peter D'Adamo, an American naturopathic doctor. The theory behind his approach was that blood types changed in different stages of our evolution – and our ability to cope with certain types of food changed as we evolved.

- **If your blood type is O** – the original hunter–gatherer – you need to eat meat and cut out wheat and most other grains. Your main health risks are ulcers and inflammatory diseases such as arthritis and you do well with vigorous exercise.
- **If your blood type is A** – the first vegetarian – you should eat a high carbohydrate, low fat diet, avoid dairy products and most meat, although you can have a little chicken. Your main risks are cancer and heart disease. You do well with gentle exercise such as yoga or golf. Meditate to deal with stress.
- **If your blood type is B** – the nomad – you should eat a varied diet, and can eat meat and dairy products. You like to be sociable when you exercise, so join walking groups, play tennis, join an exercise class. Your main health risks are chronic fatigue syndrome, multiple sclerosis and lupus.
- **If your blood type is AB** – you are rare, only 2–5 per cent of the world's population fall into this blood group as it has only evolved in the past 1,000 years. Your best diet is a combination of what blood groups A and B can eat. Calming, relaxing exercises are best. Your immune system is too friendly for comfort and you may be prone to viruses and infections.

Recommended reading: *The Eat Right Diet* by Dr Peter D'Adamo with Catherine Whitney, published by Century, 1998.

## The Hay Diet

The basis of this diet is that carbohydrates should not be eaten in the same meal as proteins and acid fruit – so no cheese and tomato sandwiches! It was devised by the American doctor William Howard Hay (1866–1940) to combat digestive problems. Hay believed that eating the two different classes of food together puts too big a strain on the digestive system.

Recommended reading: *Food Combining for Health*, by Doris Grant and Jean Joice, Thorsons, 1984

*Food Combining for Vegetarians*, by Jackie Le Tissier, Thorsons, 1992

*Raw Energy Food Combining Diet*, by Leslie Kenton, Ebury Press, 1999

## Dietary tips for a long and healthy life

1 Avoid overeating. Never eat to the point of being full. Since so much of the ageing process is concerned with processing food, within reason, the less we burden our system, the better (see the box on 'Eating less and living longer' overleaf).

2 Do not eat late at night. Eat the last meal of each day as early as possible – it should be small in size and nourishing.

3 Avoid sudden, extreme diet changes; if you are going to change your diet, do it gradually.

4 Foods should be easily digestible. Chew your food well, but if you can't chew well, use a sieve or food processor to do some of the work for you.

5 Avoid food which puts a strain on the system, particularly sugar and salt. This is tricky because as we get older, we tend to want more salt and sugar. The sense of taste can fade with age, and adding more salt and sugar seems to make food tastier.

Too much salt increases blood pressure and reduces our ability to absorb other minerals. Sugar needs to be processed by insulin which is made in the pancreas. As we get older, insulin production becomes more difficult and we may be more likely to suffer from diabetes. Both sugar and salt give us a quick lift because they go straight into the bloodstream, but anything that can give us a quick lift can also bring us down again, and when we come down, it's usually with a thump. Coffee and alcohol are notorious for this roller coaster effect. Try using more spices and less salt and for that sweet tooth, dried fruit and honey are good substitutes.

## Eating less and living longer

In the 1930s, Clive McCay at Cornell University carried out a series of experiments in which he severely restricted calories in rats, but supplied them with vitamins and mineral supplements from the time of weaning. He found that these animals lived as much as twice as long as a control group which were allowed to eat as much as they wanted.

In the 1970s, Morris Ross at the Institute for Cancer Research in Philadelphia extended the maximum life span of rats by 50–60 per cent by underfeeding them. This is the equivalent of humans living to be 170.

Source: Leslie Kenton's *Ageless Ageing*, Vermilion, 1995 – which has these references from the original papers.

McCay, Clive. *Clinical Aspects of Ageing and the Effect of Diet upon Ageing* in Cowdry's *Problems of Ageing*, 3rd ed. New York, Williams & Williams Co., 1950.

Ross, M.H. et al, *Length of life and caloric intake*, American Journal of Clinical Nutrition, August 1972, 25:834–838.

# Nutritional therapy

Nutritional therapy is the use of diet, vitamins, minerals and dietary supplements for healthy living.

## History of nutritional therapy

Dr James Lind, physician to the British Navy in the 18th century, found that sailors who were given citrus fruits were able to avoid suffering from scurvy on long sea voyages. Dr Lind's results were published in 1753, but it took another 42 years for the Navy to act on his recommendations.

At the time, no one knew why the citrus fruits prevented scurvy, but in 1928 Albert Szent-Gyorgyi isolated the active ingredient which he extracted from orange juice, cabbage juice and the adrenal glands of animals. He called it hexuronic acid because of its chemical structure. It later became known as ascorbic acid or vitamin C.

American biochemist Linus Pauling (1901–1992) made vitamin C famous. His book *Vitamin C and the Common Cold* (1970) showed that large doses of vitamin C could combat the common cold. The medical establishment was dismissive of his claims, but many people tried the vitamin C remedy and found it worked.

Pauling researched other vitamins and minerals, and called this approach orthomolecular medicine – meaning correct molecules. Pauling claimed that we can live an extra 12–18 years if we take 3–12 milligrams of Vitamin C a day, the equivalent of 45–180 oranges. He claimed that he never had a cold after he started taking vitamin C and, although he died of cancer at the age of 93, he believed that he delayed the cancer by 20 years by taking vitamin C.

Although Pauling made vitamins famous, he was not the first to use vitamins as medicine. In 1939 Dr Harvey Cleckley described dramatic success stories with large doses of vitamin B3 which helped patients with mental problems such as mania and hallucinations. In the 1950s more pioneering work was done by Dr Abraham Hoffer and Dr Humphry Osmond who had been using high doses of vitamin B3 to treat schizophrenia and claimed success rates of more than 75 per cent in 2000 cases. The use of very high doses of vitamins to combat particular illnesses is known as megavitamin therapy and, in Britain at least, it is mainly used to support the immune system in people suffering from cancer and of course, for people who want to ward off colds.

## Do you have enough vitamin C?

- Vitamin C is responsible for maintaining collagen – a protein which is necessary for making connective tissue in skin, ligaments and bones.
- Vitamin C plays an important rôle in healing wounds and burns because it helps scar tissue to form.

- It also helps form red blood cells and prevents bleeding.
- It helps the body to fight infections.

The body losses its ability to absorb vitamin C through stress, fever, long-term use of antibiotics or cortisone and aspirin. At its worst, vitamin C deficiency can result in scurvy. The symptoms of this horrible disease include:

- Sallow and muddy skin
- Lack of energy, exhaustion
- Breathlessness
- Desire to sleep most of the time
- Joint pain, particularly in the legs
- Sore gums which bleed easily
- Teeth falling out
- Brittle, easily broken bones
- Reddish skin spots
- Purple or swollen eyelids
- Nosebleeds
- Blood in urine.

In the final stages of the disease, people died of infections such as pneumonia or they collapsed after mild exertion.

Even if we do not get full blown scurvy, we may still suffer from some of the less dramatic symptoms of vitamin C deficiency such as:

- Lack of mental alertness
- Bleeding gums
- Borderline anaemia
- Irritability
- Susceptibility to infections
- Bruising

Since the 1990s there has been increasing interest in using food supplements as people became more aware that because of the way food is produced, it does not necessarily provide very much in the way of nutrition. The nutritional value of the food we eat is reduced by:

- Use of chemicals, fertilisers, pesticides, herbicides, hormones and antibodies
- Use of food additives, artificial colours, flavours, stabilising agents, sweeteners and antioxidants
- Storage – food that is eaten straight from the source is more nourishing than food that has been picked, packed, travelled and stored
- Processing and refining
- Cooking methods.

This depletion in nutrition can be minimised by using local, organically produced whole foods and by taking vitamin and mineral supplements.

How much nutrition we actually receive from the food we eat and the supplements we take depends on how efficiently we absorb the nutrients into the bloodstream. The quantity of nutrients we need varies enormously from time to time and from person to person – it may vary from individual to individual by as much as 700 per cent. This makes a nonsense of minimum standards for vitamins and minerals because what suits some people will be completely inadequate for others.

## What happens when you have a treatment?

Apart from nutritional therapists, other therapists such as naturopaths and kinesiologists may sometimes prescribe nutritional supplements as part of their treatment.

The therapist will discuss your problems and will need to find out which supplements you actually need. This may be done through iridology (looking at your eyes to diagnose your health problems) muscle testing or through laboratory analysis of your hair, urine, stools etc. Once your needs have been analysed, the therapist may suggest changes to your diet and any supplements that you need.

## Some more definitions

**RDAs – Recommended Daily Allowances** Guidelines based on expert opinions, which may differ widely from country to country.

**DRVs – Dietary Reference Values** British equivalent of RDAs which will stop nutrient deficiency diseases such as scurvy, beri-beri or pellagra, but it may not be enough for ordinary good health. Just because a particular quantity of a substance is enough to stop us getting ill, does not necessarily mean it is enough to make us healthy.

**SONAs – Suggested Optimal Nutrient Allowances** The result of a 15 year study by Dr Emanuel Cheraskin and Dr W.M. Ringsdorf. These are the suggested level of nutrients associated with optimum health.

Most of us do not even get the minimum nourishment from our food and the average diet in Britain is deficient in 7 out of 13 vitamins. This is based on the analysis of food diaries kept by 8034 households in 1993 (National Food Survey, Ministry of Agriculture, Fisheries and Food). Older people were one of the groups of people who were most likely to be eating an unhealthy diet.

## What is nutritional therapy suitable for?

Vitamin and mineral supplements have been used to treat a wide variety of illnesses, many of which are common in older people. For example:

- Cancer (vitamin C, A, beta carotene)
- Colds and infections (vitamin C)
- Allergies (vitamin C)
- Auto-immune disorders (vitamin C)
- Peripheral vascular and coronary heart disease (vitamin E)
- Cataracts (reduced risk with vitamin C and E supplements).

## ADVANTAGES OF THIS FORM OF TREATMENT

- High doses can be used without ill effects.

## DISADVANTAGES OF THIS FORM OF TREATMENT

- It can be hard to get the dose right. Too little, and it will not work and may be a waste of time and money. Too much and you may literally be pouring money down the toilet. The body takes only the vitamins it needs, the surplus is passed out of the body in the urine.

## SELF-TREATMENT

You can treat yourself with nutritional supplements, but you can waste a lot of money by buying supplements that you do not really need. If you feel that you do want to try some supplements yourself consider:

- Multi-vitamin and multi-minerals tablets
- Fish oil supplement (for vitamins A and D)
- Vitamin C
- Vitamin E
- Co-enzyme 10 (sometimes known as Q10)
- Anti-oxidant tablets, which contain a balance of vitamins A, C and E.

When you are taking any form of supplement or herbal remedy, it is a good idea to give your body a holiday from it every few months.

## Resources:

*Healing with Whole Foods* by Paul Pitchford. Published by North Atlantic Books, 1996

# 9

# Helping Yourself

## Introduction

This chapter is about what you can do to help yourself to stay as healthy as possible in body, mind, emotions and spirit. Here are some fairly simple things that you can do which can have a beneficial effect on your health and well-being.

| | |
|---|---|
| **Eat well** | This is the single most important thing you can do to help yourself. Eat at least five pieces of fruit and vegetables a day. Eat slowly, chew well and take pleasure from your food – don't eat when you are upset. |
| **Exercise** | If you are healthy go for a brisk 20 minute walk at least three times a week, if not every day. Do some form of exercise that you enjoy – whether it is walking, cycling, dancing or something else. If you are not well enough to do much in the way of exercise, do whatever you can. Ask your doctor to refer you to a physiotherapist to give you exercises that you can do. Try some of the exercises in the 'Chinese self-help' box. |
| **Get rid of clutter** | If we want our energy to flow freely it helps if our surroundings are clear and uncluttered. Getting rid of things we no longer need can be very liberating. Apart from anything else, it helps us to find things we need more easily and stops us bumping into things. |

| | |
|---|---|
| **Relax** | Do the relaxation exercise (page 216), listen to a relaxation tape or simply listen to relaxing music. |
| **Laugh** | A laugh a day keeps the doctor at bay. Like any form of relaxation, laughter is a perfect antidote to stress. |
| **Love** | Loving and being loved is as important an antidote to stress as laughter and as nourishing as food. It is one of the fundamental joys of life that makes it worth living. |

Feelings of love come from within ourselves, radiating outwards, and the therapies in this chapter help us to get in touch with our inner core. These therapies are holistic since they affect the whole of us, even if this is not immediately obvious.

- **Yoga** and **T'ai chi** focus on the body, but they also have a powerful effect on our mind, emotions and spirit.
- **The Alexander Technique** and the **better eyesight techniques** may seem as if they are purely focused on the physical body. In practice, the Alexander Technique has a profound effect on the way we stand and move in the world and how we feel about ourselves and what we do. Similarly the eyesight techniques not only change our eyesight but also the way we see ourselves and the world around us.
- **Meditation** may appear to be focused on the mind, emotions and spirit, but research shows that it can also have profound physical effects as well.

# Chinese self-help

John Brazier, Principal of the Academy of Oriental Medicine, suggests some simple exercises that anyone can do sitting in a chair.

### Throat and face stretch

- Stretch the throat by lifting the throat up.
- Stick your chin out and stretch the whole of the bottom of the neck.
- Smile as broadly as you can and exercise all the facial muscles.

When muscles stop being used, or are not used very much, they become flaccid, wrinkle and dry up. Using the muscles helps them to remember what they used to feel like when they were younger. It also helps the blood to flow and flushes out toxins.

### Ear pulls

Use your thumb and forefinger to gently pinch the outside of your ears, pulling your ears out, and gently unrolling the creases in your ears all the way from the top to the bottom of your ear lobe. Repeat five to ten times so that your ears feel hot because all the blood has rushed there.

In Chinese medicine, the entire body can be affected by what happens in the ears. Just as auricular acupuncture (ear acupuncture) affects the whole body, so this simple massage can also have an all over effect.

### Eye exercise

Roll your eyes so they make a sideways figure of eight (the symbol of infinity). Do this in both directions five to ten times.

This is good for the whole body because the eyes have muscles which are attached to the cranial bones which are in contact with every other part of the body, and this massages the cranial system (see the section on 'Cranial osteopathy', page 94).

**Tongue exercise**

Stick your tongue out of your mouth, stick it down as far as you can, then right, up, left and down in a circle. Do it one way and then the other way. Bring your tongue inside the mouth and rub it inside and outside the gums. You will probably find that this makes your mouth water.

This exercise stimulates the saliva glands in the mouth, which are important for digesting food. It also stimulates the blood flow to the teeth and gums and keeps them strong and healthy.

**Pat the organs**

Warm your hands and gently pat your organs, particularly your kidneys (on either side of your lower back) – you may find it easier if you lean forward, or do it with a friend.

This stimulates the organs by giving them more energy.

# T'ai chi and Chi gong

T'ai chi is an abbreviation of T'ai chi chuan. Both T'ai chi and Chi gong are elegant, graceful forms of moving meditation that can be used for healing and preventative medicine.

T'ai chi chuan means 'supreme, ultimate fist'. T'ai chi can also mean 'wholeness', chuan can also mean 'way' or 'method'. Chi gong means 'cultivating chi, or energy'.

## History of Chi gong and T'ai chi

Chi gong is part of traditional Chinese medicine. Some authorities say there are as many as 10,000 different ways in which Chi gong can be performed – which is not surprising as there are many different ways of cultivating chi or energy. Different forms of Chi gong include spontaneous Chi gong, which is just allowing the body to move in whatever way it wants to, Lulu Daoyin which is spontaneous natural dance to music, breathing and singing exercises, medical Chi gong which uses specific exercises to cure particular illnesses – and T'ai chi chuan.

T'ai chi chuan was developed by a Chinese Taoist monk called Chang San-feng in the 13th century AD. According to legend, he was watching a crane attack a snake and was impressed by the circular, spiralling movements the snake made as it yielded to the strong direct blows of the crane's long bill. Because the snake yielded, the crane could not use its direct force.

Chang was fascinated by these circular movements and the principles of softness and flexibility overcoming hardness and rigidity and this became the essence of T'ai chi. Chang also became interested in the graceful movements of other animals and this shows in the names of different T'ai chi movements – for example, 'stork crooks its wings', 'snake creeps down', 'embrace tiger', 'return to mountain' and so on.

Chang added these natural, circular movements, emphasising breathing and softness to a traditional form of martial art known as Shao-lin which was originally developed as a method of self-defence for monks in the 6th century AD. Today, its martial arts roots are barely visible as it is used mainly as a moving meditation and as a form of gentle exercise. Millions of Chinese people practice it in the early mornings and early evenings in parks and open spaces.

T'ai chi has been practised in Britain since the beginning of the 20th century, but it became much more popular after US President Richard Nixon visited China in 1972. World wide television audiences saw hundreds of people practising T'ai chi wherever President Nixon went. People wanted to know more about this graceful form of exercise which seemed to be enjoyed by old and young alike.

## What happens in a T'ai chi class?

It is a good idea to wear light, loose-fitting shirts and trousers and wear socks or thin slippers rather than heavy shoes. If the floor is not too cold, then it is best to have bare feet. You will be taught the movements partly by following what the teacher is doing, and partly by the teacher helping you. All the movements are performed slowly, with an awareness of exactly what you are doing.

The movements are slow, and you need to relax into the different postures. They are very simple and easy to learn, but it can take a lifetime of practice to perfect them. The movements are designed to be equally balanced between passive, gentle, yielding, flexible, feminine movements (yin) and active, strong, rooted, dynamic, masculine movements (yang) to help you get a feeling of overall balance. You will probably be told that T'ai chi is a therapy which unfolds its benefits gradually, but most people find it helps them to feel more relaxed and balanced right from their very first class.

There are two forms of T'ai chi: the long form and the short form. The short form takes about 5 to 10 minutes, while the long form has more than 100 movements and takes between 20 and 40 minutes. The whole class lasts about an hour or an hour and a half and you should feel pleasantly relaxed after a class. It can feel as if you have given yourself a powerful, internal massage.

## What is T'ai chi suitable for?

The traditional Chinese medicine way of looking at disease is to see it as a disturbance in energy or chi which may be moving too quickly or too slowly with too much energy gathering in one particular area and too little elsewhere. T'ai chi can correct these kinds of imbalances by moving the energy so that it is evenly distributed.

It can help with anxiety and stress-related conditions as it encourages relaxation, which makes it a good alternative to tranquillisers. It can also help improve breathing and posture and can generally tone up the body and stimulate circulation as well as improve body awareness, balance and confidence.

T'ai chi can also help us with the way we deal with daily life, seeing where we use unnecessary force which can cause stress and tiredness. This does not just apply to physical force, it can also help us understand our emotions and the way we relate to ourselves and others.

### ADVANTAGES OF THIS FORM OF TREATMENT

- You feel that you are doing something positive to improve your health. It is suitable for any age, and modified forms can be done even if you are not very active physically.
- It is a beautiful, enjoyable way of moving. People find it physically, mentally and spiritually rewarding.
- It can be a sociable thing to do as you take classes with other people.

## DISADVANTAGES OF THIS FORM OF TREATMENT

- It is not a 'get well quick' therapy and it takes a certain amount of patience, commitment and perseverance.
- You need to go to classes for an hour and a half every week and practice on your own in between times.

## SELF-TREATMENT

Although it is a good idea to practise between lessons, it is important to go to classes as well. This is because you need to make sure that your body is in the right positions, so that your teacher can check that you are keeping your spine vertical, your hips level and your head upright.

## Animals

Animal symbols have been an important part of Taoist philosophy since 300 AD. These include the tiger (symbol of the ego) which had to be ridden or mastered, the monkey (symbol of mischieviousness) which had to be resisted as well as the bear, the stag, the crane and others.

## Resources

*T'ai chi Ch'uan* by Chen Man Ch'ing (North Atlantic Books, 1991) describes how the author was often ill in his youth and practising T'ai chi cured him. Each time he was lazy and didn't practice he got ill again!

# Yoga

Yoga is a Sanskrit word which means 'to yoke', or 'to have union with the highest form of God', and it aims to bring balance to body, mind and spirit. The ultimate aim of yoga is enlightenment, but in Britain it is mainly taught as a combination of physical exercise and relaxation techniques.

There are many different types of yoga, including:

- Strong physical exercise
- Gentle physical exercise
- Breathing techniques
- Meditation
- Sound and chanting
- Philosophy.

## History of yoga

Yoga started in India about 4,000 years ago and there are references to yoga in the ancient Indian vedic texts. The original source of the positions and exercises are thought to be copied from the way animals seem to move and relax so much more easily than humans. It is part of the Ayurvedic system of medicine, but it is also a complete form of medicine in its own right.

For centuries yoga was practised by a few dedicated yogi philosophers and meditators who lived far away from normal civilisation. Sometimes they practised completely on their own, sometimes in small groups and they passed on their knowledge to just a handful of followers. It was only in the 20th century that yoga became available to a wider public and now it is so widespread in India that physical yoga exercises are taught in schools.

It was first brought to the West at the beginning of the 20th century and became more popular in the 1950s when various Indian teachers came to Britain. In the 1960s, John Lennon and the other Beatles discovered the Maharishi Mahesh Yogi, bringing the meditation side of yoga to public awareness. The therapeutic side of yoga was given a boost by virtuoso violinist Sir Yehudi Menuhin who cured his frozen shoulder with the help of his yoga teacher BKS Iyenkar.

In the 1990s there was a great explosion of interest in yoga as people became increasingly enthusiastic about finding natural ways of dealing with stress. Now there are yoga classes in practically every village hall and community centre, with about half a million people in Britain practising yoga regularly.

# What happens in a yoga session?

## ONE TO ONE TREATMENT

Your physical difficulties will be assessed and you will be taught a series of positions, breathing and meditation techniques which will be specially chosen to help with your particular problems.

## CLASSES

You will be taught a series of exercises that aim to stretch and release tension from the whole body. The aim of the exercises is to improve your general health and flexibility and also help your endocrine system, lymphatic system and immune system. If you have health problems, you should go to an experienced remedial yoga teacher.

The movements are done slowly and the postures held for a minute or more to help you become aware of your body, its tensions and the way it behaves. At the end of the class you may learn meditation, relaxation or breathing techniques to quieten the mind. You may also be taught recuperative poses which are particularly relaxing positions. A class usually lasts for about an hour and a half. It is a good idea to go at least once a week and to practice in between classes.

There are many different types of yoga and it is important to find one that suits you and your level of fitness. The most common form of yoga in Britain is known as Hatha yoga, which consists of physical exercises, breathing exercises and meditation. Hatha yoga comes in several different styles, and it can be practised in many different ways. It is important to choose the style that suits your own needs and, preferably, a teacher with whom you feel comfortable.

Other forms of yoga include:

**Karma yoga**  Trying to undo the sins of your past lives so that you do not carry them into the next.

**Yantra yoga**  Meditating on different symbols to discover who you are. The symbols represent different soul states.

**Mantra yoga** Making sounds to purify the body. This is the basis for Transcendental Meditation (see the section on 'Meditation' later in this chapter).

**Tantra yoga**   Rising above your physical desires by completely indulging in them according to very strict rules.

**Raja yoga**   The 'yoga of kings' which is based on the philosophy of the ancient texts.

The ultimate aim of yoga is to achieve enlightenment and even those varieties which seem to be very physical are also concerned with keeping the energy body healthy. The idea is to purify the body so that the spirit can be liberated. The main energy channel is believed to run up and down the spine, with smaller channels called Nadis running off the main channel.

In the yoga tradition, the health of our energy system is maintained by the chakras or seven wheels of energy which are positioned on the spine. Indeed, there is a yoga saying, 'You are only as old as your spine'.

## What is yoga suitable for?

Yoga strengthens areas where there is weakness, which is useful for problems such as weak backs. It also releases areas where there is tension, making it helpful for stress-related conditions.

When you are thinking about what kind of yoga to try, it is important to bear in mind your age, how flexible you are, your level of physical fitness and your temperament. When you are choosing a yoga class think about what you really need. If you are normally physically active, you may feel you want a very active form of yoga, but a relaxing class may have a more balancing effect. Similarly if you don't normally take much exercise, you may find it helpful to go to a more active class.

Yoga is particularly good for:

- Angina and other heart problems
- Arthritis
- Asthma
- Back problems
- Co-ordination problems
- Hypertension and other stress-related conditions

- Insomnia
- Multiple sclerosis
- Mental problems
- Stiffness.

If you suffer from asthma or angina, practising some of the relaxation techniques can be particularly helpful.

## Investigating the effectiveness of yoga

The Yoga Biomedical Trust conducted a poll of 2700 people who practised yoga and were suffering from one or more of 20 complaints. For each condition over 70 per cent said that yoga had helped them to improve.

- Back pain – out of 1142 people, 98 per cent were helped
- Arthritis and rheumatism – 589 people, 90 per cent were helped
- Anxiety – 838 people, 94 per cent were helped
- Insomnia – 542 people, 82 per cent were helped
- Nerve or muscle disease – 112 people, 96 per cent were helped
- Hypertension – 150 people, 84 per cent were helped
- Heart disease – 50 people, 94 per cent were helped
- Obesity – 240 people, 74 per cent were helped
- Diabetes – 10 people, 80 per cent were helped
- Cancer – 29 people, 90 per cent were helped

(Source: *Reader's Digest Family Guide to Alternative Medicine*, poll conducted in 1983)

### ADVANTAGES OF THIS FORM OF TREATMENT

- Yoga is a self-help form of therapy and enables you to take responsibility for your own well-being.
- Once you have learned yoga, you can practise it at home without any extra cost.
- It can be a sociable activity if you want to do it in a class with a group of people.
- Advocates of yoga say that it delays ageing and helps you grow old gracefully. If practised under proper supervision, it can be a gentle

form of exercise which doesn't put a strain on the joints or force you to use too much oxygen.

- You can exercise as vigorously or as gently as you want.

### DISADVANTAGES OF THIS FORM OF TREATMENT

- It is not a 'get well quick' technique. It takes time – time to learn the postures and time to practise them.
- It can cause joint strain if you are over-enthusiastic with the postures.
- If you are unfit or ill, or find it difficult to lie on the floor, it can be difficult to find the right teacher who can adapt the exercises to suit you.

### SELF-TREATMENT

Although you can learn yoga from videos, tapes and books, it is best to learn from an experienced, qualified teacher – at least in the beginning.

# Meditation

The word 'meditate' comes from the Sanskrit word for 'wisdom'. It is a way of being in a focused, attentive, yet relaxed state.

## History of meditation

Meditation has been an important part of all the major religions – just as prayer is talking to God, meditation is listening to God. In the Jewish and Christian religions it has largely taken the form of contemplation, or thinking about the Divine, while in the Eastern religions, the emphasis is on emptying the mind.

In the 1960s the Maharishi Mahesh Yogi introduced Transcendental Meditation (TM) to the west and there was a general surge of interest in meditation techniques. The Maharishi claimed that meditation made people healthier because it could lower blood pressure and help the heart and lungs work more efficiently. It produced what Professor Herbert Benson called 'The Relaxation Response'. Since the 1960s, over 600 studies have shown that Transcendental Meditation really does help with stress-related problems such as high blood pressure, heart disease, anxiety and depression.

Transcendental Meditation is the brand name for a particular form of meditation where you are taught to repeat a single word (known as a mantra) over and over again. There are many other forms of meditation which have been described in books and practised in groups all over Britain.

## What happens during meditation?

Meditation is not a treatment, but a practice – something you do every day as part of your spiritual journey, although you may also be doing it to improve your health.

- If possible, sit in an upright chair with your back straight, or sit on the floor with your back straight and legs crossed (if you practise yoga, you may want to sit in the lotus position). The exact position you choose does not really matter – what does matter is that your back should be straight and you should feel comfortable. It is not a good idea to meditate lying down as you will probably fall asleep.
- Choose a time and place where you will not be disturbed.
- Remember that it takes time and energy to change from an ordinary state of consciousness to the relaxed but alert state of meditative consciousness. Allow yourself time at the end of the meditation to return gently to 'normal'. You may find it helpful to stretch, or simply become aware of yourself sitting on the chair (or on the ground) and the room around you, before you open your eyes.

Some of the more common forms of meditation include the following.

### ATTENTION TO THE BREATH

Breathing is a link between the body and the mind. When you feel calm, your breathing is naturally deep and slow, but if you have a fright, you automatically catch your breath, and if you are generally tense, anxious or upset, your breathing tends to be faster and more shallow. Relaxed breathing should come from your belly, not your upper chest.

To see what is happening with your own breathing, put one hand just below your collarbone, with the other hand on your abdomen, just below your belly button. Breathe naturally and see which hand rises and falls with your breathing. When you are fully relaxed, only the hand that is on your abdomen will move. If the hand on your abdomen isn't moving at all, just leave your hands in the same position for a few minutes, focus on your breathing and see what happens.

There are many ways of paying attention to the breath, such as counting how long it takes to breathe in and out, or simply noticing the breath as it comes in and out of the nose.

One of the most common forms of meditation is counting the breath. Breathe in (one), breathe out, breathe in (two), breathe out, breathe in (three) etc until you reach ten and then repeat the process. If a distracting thought occurs, start again from one.

## MANTRAS

This is where you repeat a single word or several words over and over again. TM uses this technique, but it is also part of the spiritual practice of several Eastern religions. For example, the Nichiren Diashonin Buddhists repeat the words 'Nam-myoho-renge-kyo' as part of their practise. Spiritual mantras include the word 'Om' (aum) or the phrase 'Om Mani Padme Hum'. The words are usually said out loud, although in TM the words are thought rather than spoken.

## FOCUSING ON AN OBJECT

This is where you gaze at a lighted candle, a picture or abstract design (mandala) or a natural object such as a flower or a stone. This is sometimes known as 'one pointed contemplation'.

## GUIDED MEDITATION

This is where you listen to someone else who talks you through a form of meditation which usually includes a relaxation process followed by an invitation to imagine a relaxing scene such as a pool of water or a pleasant field or pasture.

Guided meditations can also be used to help you get in touch with yourself at a deep, inner level (see the section on 'Guided imagery, page 175).

## LISTENING

Listening to the sound of ocean waves, waterfalls or birds can put you in a relaxed, meditative state, but it is not really a meditation practice as such.

## MINDFULNESS

This is where you are totally focused and aware of what is happening to you and your surroundings.

When we are in pain, it is natural to become tense and try to resist what is happening to us and we probably imagine and magnify the danger and the misery of it all. If you use mindfulness, you don't resist the pain, but pay very close attention to it, discovering what particular qualities it has, whether it is sharp or dull, what shape, colour, and intensity it has. You are not trying to change anything, just allowing the pain to be whatever it wants to be. It may feel unnatural because it is the opposite of what we normally do, but with practice you may find that it is less painful to accept the pain than to resist it. The pain may not go away completely, but it may be substantially reduced.

## What is meditation suitable for?

Meditation can be used in several ways. For example:

- As a spiritual practice – a way of listening to the Divine.
- As a relaxing antidote to stress and stress-related illnesses such as high blood pressure.
- It is particularly helpful for people with insomnia.
- As a way of changing consciousness for pain relief.
- As a route to personal growth.

### ADVANTAGES OF THIS FORM OF TREATMENT

- It is something that you can do to help yourself.
- It can help to put you in touch with who you really are.

### DISADVANTAGES OF THIS FORM OF TREATMENT

- It takes time, commitment and patience. Although it sounds easy, it isn't.

- It also takes energy to change from one state of consciousness to another. If you are ill and have very little energy, it is probably better to use relaxation techniques instead.

## SELF-TREATMENT

This therapy is suitable for treating yourself – no one can do it for you. But it is hard to do it on your own, so it helps to have a meditation teacher or join a meditation group. Books can also be helpful.

### Resources

*Moon Over Water*, by Jessica Macbeth. Published by Gateway Books, 1990.

# Relaxation

There is a link between warmth and heaviness and feelings of deep relaxation. Hypnotherapists sometimes suggest feelings of warmth and heaviness as part of what is known as the induction process when they help you to enter the hypnotic state.

But you can create this feeling of deep relaxation for yourself, simply by telling yourself that each part of your body is warm and heavy.

You can start by saying to yourself: 'My left hand is feeling warm and heavy. My forearm is feeling warm and heavy ...' and so on with all the different parts of your body.

It can be particularly helpful for people who suffer from high blood pressure and other stress-related problems. The problem with stress is that we are not always aware that we are suffering from it, which is where biofeedback can be helpful (see the section on Biofeedback, page 218).

One of the telltale signs of stress is cold hands and feet. Some people who suffer from migraine find that if they can imagine that their hands are warm at the first suspicion that they may be getting a migraine, they can sometimes stop it happening altogether.

# Relaxation exercise

You may find it helpful to record this and play it to yourself until you know what to do by heart.

- Sit in a comfortable chair with your back straight. If this isn't possible, sit with your back as straight as you can, or lie down with your back as straight as possible.
- The difficulty with lying down is that it increases the chances of you falling asleep – but that is not such a terrible thing, if the aim is to be as relaxed as possible.
- Start by taking a couple of deep breaths. Breathe in peace, breathe out anything you don't want or need. Breathe in peace, breathe out anything you don't want or need.
- Pay attention to your breathing, there's no need to change it, just be aware of your breath.
- Now focus on your feet. Imagine that they are warm and heavy.
- Your feet are warm and heavy.
- Now imagine that the warmth and heaviness in your feet is rising up through your legs, up through your calves to your knees, so that from your knees to your feet, you feel warm and heavy.
- Feel that from your knees to your feet, you feel warm and heavy.
- Now imagine that the warmth and heaviness in your feet and your legs is spreading higher up your legs to your hips, so that from your hips to your knees, and from your knees to your feet, you feel warm and heavy.
- Feel that from your hips to your knees and feet, you feel warm and heavy.
- Now imagine that the warmth and heaviness in your feet and your legs is spreading up past your hips to your stomach, so that your stomach feels warm and heavy, so that from your stomach to your hips, and right down to your feet, you feel warm and heavy.
- Feel that from your stomach to your legs, and right down to your feet, you feel warm and heavy.
- Now imagine that the warmth and heaviness in your stomach is spreading right up through your body, so that from your shoulders to your stomach, to your legs and right down to your feet, you feel warm and heavy.

- Feel that your entire body, from your shoulders to your hips and down your legs to your feet, feels warm and heavy.
- Now imagine that the warmth and heaviness in your shoulders is going down your arms to your hands and fingers, which now feel warm and heavy, so that your shoulders and arms and hands, and your whole body right down to your legs and feet, are warm and heavy.
- Feel that your hands and arms and your entire body, from your shoulders to your hips and down your legs to your feet feels warm and heavy.
- Now imagine that the warmth and heaviness in your shoulders is going down your back, melting any tightness in your shoulders and the back of the neck, so that your entire body from your shoulders to your arms and hands, and your entire body down to your legs and feet, feels warm and heavy.
- Feel that your entire body, from your shoulders to your arms and hands, and your entire body down to your legs and feet, feels warm and heavy.
- Now feel the warmth and heaviness spreading up your neck until the warmth and heaviness spreads to your whole face, so that you feel warmth and heaviness in your face, particularly around your mouth and jaw, and your eyes, so that your face, neck and body right down to your legs and feet feel warm and heavy.
- Feel that your face and neck and your entire body, from your shoulders to your arms and hands, and right down to your legs and feet, feel warm and heavy.
- Now feel the warmth and heaviness spreading over your fore-head and scalp, so that the warmth and heaviness is now covering you from the very top of your head, down through your head and neck and shoulders to your arms and hands, and right down to your legs and feet, so that your entire body feels warm and heavy.
- Feel that the warmth and heaviness is now covering you from the very top of your head, so that your entire body, down through your head and neck and shoulders to your arms and hands, and right down to your legs and feet, feels warm and heavy.

- Enjoy feeling that warmth and heaviness throughout your whole body for as long as you want to.
- When you are ready, take a couple of deep breaths, be aware of the room around you, stretch your fingers and toes and slowly and gradually in your own time, open your eyes.

# Biofeedback

Children learn by immediate, natural and sometimes painful feedback. When they are learning to walk, they fall over a lot until they get the hang of it. Learning by our mistakes and getting feedback is the way we learn to do almost everything. Biofeedback tells us what the body is doing, so that we can learn to control it.

## How biofeedback works

We don't always know that what we're doing is hurting us. For example, if we feel hot and headachy, we may need to use a thermometer to tell us that we have got a temperature and should stop what we are doing and go to bed. When we have high blood pressure, we may not even be aware of the problem until the doctor measures it for us.

Biofeedback uses instruments that tell us what is going on inside our bodies, so that we can change it. It was first used in America in the 1970s on laboratory monkeys and rats who learned to reduce their blood pressure without affecting their heart rate, and to reduce their heart rate without affecting their blood pressure. Today, biofeedback is used by people who work out in gyms. They use wrist monitors to measure heart and pulse rates so that they can work within safe limits. There are also biofeedback machines that can show you how relaxed you are, which is useful if you want to control your blood pressure. Biofeedback machines can also help with migraines and urinary incontinence.

The idea behind biofeedback is the same, regardless of what it is used for. The instruments give you information about what is happening in your body – if you want to change what is happening, then you have to learn how. This may mean learning how to relax, or learning muscle control, it all depends on what you use the machines for.

# The Alexander Technique

This technique teaches you how to use your body in a way that is stress-free and effortless.

## History of the Alexander Technique

The Alexander Technique is named after its inventor, Frederick Matthias Alexander, an Australian actor who lost his voice and, as a result, discovered a new way of standing, walking, sitting and lying down.

Alexander had been a successful actor until he started losing his voice. He would recover after resting, but he lost his voice again when he went back to work. He realised that he must be doing something wrong when he was acting, and he studied himself in the mirror to try and find out exactly what it was. In this way, he discovered that when he started to say his lines, he would pull his head back, push his chest out and this would put pressure on his vocal cords, tighten his breathing and create tension throughout his body. No wonder he could barely talk. By looking at himself in the mirror, he taught himself to relax into more natural, comfortable positions. His breathing improved and so did his voice. It took ten years to perfect what became known as 'the Alexander Technique' and, although Alexander returned to the stage, he soon became better known for his technique than his acting.

Other actors flocked to him, wanting to learn his new technique, and when he came to London in 1905 well known personalities such as the writers Aldous Huxley and George Bernard Shaw came to him for lessons. Alexander also lived in America which helped the technique to gain an international reputation.

Alexander had a severe stroke and lost the use of his left arm and leg when he was 78. But he used the technique and regained the use of his body and all his faculties and lived for another eight years.

## What happens when you have a lesson in the Alexander Technique?

The basic idea behind the technique is to encourage you to replace your normal stress patterns with more relaxing ways of using your body. At your first lesson, the teacher will probably ask about any health problems you may have, but they will focus on looking at you and how you move, stand and sit. They will also feel what you are doing by placing their hands gently on your neck, shoulders and back. This shows them how you 'use' your body.

It is a good idea to wear comfortable clothes for the lesson, and women will probably find it helpful to wear trousers rather than a skirt.

You will probably be asked to perform some simple movements – walking, standing up or sitting down in a chair, while the teacher's hands stay in contact with your body. While the teacher is learning about how you move, they are also gently guiding your body, encouraging you to release muscle tension. Like any other teacher, they vary in their approach according to their personality and training. Some teachers may talk and explain what they are doing; others prefer to spend the first lesson helping you to get a new experience of ease and flexibility. You will be asked to be aware of three suggestions:

- That the neck be free
- That the head move forward and upward, so that
- The back lengthens and widens.

It is natural to fall into your normal stress patterns and it takes a conscious effort to change – to stop your unconscious habits and replace them with more useful conscious ways of being. The lesson will often end with some work that is done lying down on a massage couch. Your head is usually placed on a pile of books and your feet are placed on the couch with your knees up. This position ensures that your whole back is on the table. It feels very relaxing, particularly when the teacher adjusts your body and touches you, encouraging your body to follows the suggestions that your neck be free and that your back lengthens and widens.

A lesson usually lasts between 30 and 45 minutes, although it can take as long as an hour. Exactly how many lessons you have will depend partly on how many you need, and how many you can afford. You may get some benefit from a single lesson, but of course, the more lessons you have, the more you will learn.

It is usually a good idea to work quite intensively (at least once or twice a week) for a few months. Once you have got the hang of the technique you can come back for refresher lessons every few weeks or months. Some Alexander teachers also offer group work where several people learn the technique at the same time.

## What is the Alexander Technique suitable for?

The technique is helpful for any problems which are made worse by tension in the back of the neck – so it can he helpful for chronic back problems, arthritis, headaches, and migraines.

### ADVANTAGES OF THIS FORM OF TREATMENT

- It is something you can do for yourself.
- It not only helps you with existing problems, but helps you avoid problems in the future.
- It is not strenuous or difficult.
- It helps you learn about your body and how you use it.
- There is no need to take your clothes off.
- It can undo bad habits that have taken a lifetime to create.
- Once you've learned it, the benefits can last a lifetime.

### DISADVANTAGES OF THIS FORM OF TREATMENT

- It takes time and commitment to practice.

### SELF-TREATMENT

Practising the Alexander Technique is obviously an important part of the process, but actually learning the technique on your own is very difficult. Alexander himself used to say: 'Anyone can do what I did, if they will do what I did'. But few people want to spend ten years following in his footsteps and by the end of his life Alexander realised that attempts to put his teaching into practice without the help of a teacher were seldom successful.

## *Try it yourself*

One of the basic ideas behind the Alexander Technique is that your body follows instructions from your mind.

Try getting up off your chair:

- What does it feel like if you think 'up'?
- What does it feel like if you think 'down'?

If you use a walking stick, instead of thinking down to the stick, imagine that you are like a flower, rising up above the stick.

## *Resources*

*The Use of the Self*, by F Matthias Alexander. Reissued by Gollancz, 1986

*How to Learn the Alexander Technique – A manual for students*. By Barbara and William Conable, Andover Road Publishers, 1992

*Alternative Health: Alexander Technique*, by C. Stevens. Optima, 1987

# Better eyesight without glasses

This section describes a method of learning how to improve your eyesight without lenses or surgery.

## *History of the method*

The Bates method of improving your eyesight was devised by New York eye specialist Dr William H Bates (1860–1931) after observing many thousands of people with eye problems. He found that:

- Normal sight is naturally changeable – we see more clearly if we are relaxed and interested, but it is harder to see if we are tense, bored or worried.
- Some eye problems will change without treatment – some will obviously get worse, but they can also get better.
- Many patients complained of eyestrain and headaches, even though they had responded well to medical treatment.

Bates believed that we did not see with our eyes alone, but with our whole selves – mind, body, and spirit. He thought that poor sight can be the result of an underlying health problem and/or the result of bad habits which may date back to childhood. He found that people often felt tense and anxious about seeing and that learning a more relaxed approach could actually improve their vision.

In 1919 Bates wrote his book *The Cure of Imperfect Eyesight*, which is still in print under the more modest title *Better Eyesight without Glasses*. Today, there are Bates Method teachers in the US and England and a number of self-help books which are based on his technique.

## What happens when you have a treatment?

Like many other complementary therapists, the Bates practitioner will ask you questions about your health and lifestyle. They will also ask about any problems you have had in the past, such as whether you:

- Have had any accidents, particularly head injuries.
- Suffer from headaches, migraines or any other health problems and are taking any medication.

They will also want to know about your eyes. It is a good idea to bring your glasses, and if you have a copy of your prescription or any medical reports, bring these too. If you wear contact lenses be prepared to take them out, so bring your lenses holder.

The next stage is for the Bates practitioner to test your eyes to see how well you can see without glasses or contact lenses. This is called a vision assessment, which consists of a number of eye tests including the eye chart that opticians use. You will be encouraged to relax, and the idea behind the assessment is to find out how well your eyes work. At this point the Bates practitioner will have a reasonable idea about what you need to do in order to improve your eyesight, and will discuss this with you.

At the end of the first session you will be given some simple exercises to practice which will help you to start to experience relaxing your eyes and thinking about the whole process of perception. These sessions should not replace regular eye testing by an optician, which is particularly important as you get older. The Bates method is not so much a treatment, more a lesson in how to use your eyes without strain. Sessions usually last about an hour and most people need about 6–10 weekly sessions.

## Aldous Huxley

The writer Aldous Huxley had always had bad eyesight and needed thick magnifying glasses to read. In 1939, when he was 45 years old, he was losing his eyesight, but within two months of starting the Bates exercises, he was able to read without glasses. He wrote a book called *The Art of Seeing* which describes his experience.

## What is this method suitable for?

The Bates method is particularly suited to people who want to stop their eyesight deteriorating as they get older. Bates enthusiasts say that it can help anyone improve their eyes in some way, and you are never too old to learn.

### CATARACTS

This is the name given to any complaint where the lens of the eye loses its transparency. It can be caused by inflexibility in the use of the eye. Cataracts are often associated with diabetes, and the incidence tends to be higher among people who are on long-term steroid use. The Bates method, which encourages relaxed, flexible action, may be worth trying while waiting for an operation. It may also be helpful to have homeopathic treatment.

### GLAUCOMA

Glaucoma is raised pressure in the eye. Acute glaucoma is always a medical emergency, but if chronic glaucoma is diagnosed in its early stages, the Bates method is well worth trying.

### ADVANTAGES OF THIS FORM OF TREATMENT

- Once you have learned the exercises you can do them on your own.
- It can save you money on glasses and contact lenses.
- It can change more than just the way you see things, it can change the way you perceive and understand aspects of yourself and the world around you.

### DISADVANTAGES OF THIS FORM OF TREATMENT

- It takes time, patience and perseverance.

### SELF-TREATMENT

This therapy is suitable for treating yourself. In fact you have to treat yourself – no one can do the exercises for you. But it is important to see a Bates practitioner as well, so that you know that you are doing the right exercises for your particular condition, and you are doing them in the right way.

Both the Bates method and the Alexander Technique are concerned with re-training, helping you to stop doing what comes automatically and start doing something else, something that is more helpful than your normal habits. This means you really do need a teacher who can tell you that although what you are doing may feel wrong, it is actually right.

## Tips for making the most of your eyesight

- Read in a good light, blink often and look up briefly at the end of every page.
- Rest your eyes when using VDUs for one minute in every twelve. If possible, put your hands in front of your eyes (palming technique).
- Do not do anything which hurts your eyes or blurs your vision, such as watching a lot of television in the dark.
- Get your eyes tested regularly.

## Better eyesight exercises

It is important to practice the exercises regularly, and relax when you do them. Your eyes can't relax if your neck and shoulders are tense. Do not overwork or strain your eyes when you are doing the exercises. Do not try to do too much, too quickly, do not try all the exercises at once.

### 1 Palming

Sit in a comfortable, relaxed position at a desk or table. Close your eyes and rest your elbows on a cushion on the table, keeping your back and neck straight and your head level. Cover your eyes without touching them with your cupped palms. Now think of something you enjoy, imagine your favourite flowers, remember a favourite holiday or listen to some relaxing music while you sit with your hands cupped over your eyes for ten minutes.

While palming your eyes, you can try to remember something in vivid detail with bright colours. According to Bates, remembering something in your mind's eye helps you to see things more clearly in reality. Relax, and don't strain yourself.

### 2 Shifting

Move your gaze from one point of interest to another.

### 3 Blinking

Get into the habit of blinking regularly once or twice every ten seconds to clean and lubricate the eyes.

### 4 Near and far focusing

Hold two pencils or your index fingers in front of your face. One pencil or finger should be about three inches (75 mm) away, the other should be held at arm's length. Focus on one finger or pencil with both eyes, then blink and focus on the other. Repeat this several times whenever you can.

## 5 Splashing

First thing every morning splash your closed eyes 20 times with warm water and then 20 times with cold water to stimulate the circulation. Last thing at night, splash with cold water first, and then warm water.

## 6 Swinging

Stand with your feet apart and sway gently from side to side, letting your eyes swing along with your body's movement. Be aware of the visual movement as this relaxes your eyes and helps them to become more flexible. Repeat whenever you get a chance and you may find it helpful to play music while doing this exercise.

## *Other forms of eye exercises*

Bates' ideas were based on personal experience, but they use many of the techniques which are recognised in traditional forms of natural medicine such as Ayurvedic medicine (yoga) and naturopathic medicine (hydrotherapy).

### YOGA EYE EXERCISES (NETRA VYAAYAMAM)

- Take off your glasses and contact lenses.
- Sit up straight, with your shoulders relaxed and the chest comfortable and expanded.
- Breathe allowing the abdomen to soften so the lungs can take a deep breath in, then breathe out, contracting the abdomen as the air leaves through the nostrils. Relax the breath and the face.
- With your eyes open, eyelids relaxed and gaze soft, keep your head still, but move the eyes up and down, following an imaginary line from floor to ceiling. Do this several times without straining the eyes.
- Close your eyes for long enough to relax.
- With your eyes open, eyelids relaxed and gaze soft, keep your head still, but move your eyes as far to the right as possible, keeping your head relaxed and centred.

- Now move your eyes along an imaginary horizontal line to the far left, try not to let your eyes dip downwards. Do this several times without straining.
- Close your eyes for long enough to relax them.
- Open your eyes, let them soften, then look up as far as you can, keeping your head centred. Then trace an imaginary circle with the eyes by gently moving them to the right, then down, then smoothly to the far left and up again. Do this several times without straining.
- Close your eyes for long enough to relax them.

## Resources

*The Bates Method*, by Peter Mansfield. Published by Vermilion, 1995

*The Art of Seeing* by Aldous Huxley, Chatto & Windus, 1941

*Meir Schneider's Miracle Eyesight Method: The Natural Way to Heal and Improve your Vision*. Available on Sounds True (Audiocassette), 1997

Meir Schneider was born blind, but he was determined to learn how to see. He began his own intensive exploration of sight and self-healing systems which included the Bates method.

# SECTION 3

# 10

# Where to Go for Help

If you have turned to this section, you are at least toying with the idea of trying one of the complementary therapies. Once you have actually made the decision to go ahead, you are making the first step in finding the right therapy and therapist. By choosing complementary therapy, you are supporting your own vital force, your own natural ability to heal yourself. Once you have made that decision, that same natural ability to heal yourself will help you to find the most appropriate therapy and therapist.

While there are some logical steps you can take to find the right kind of help, be prepared for luck and happy coincidences to play their part. You may find that three people recommend the same therapist to you – or that bus drivers and strangers start talking about a particular therapy. When this kind of thing happens – as it will – pay attention and follow the clues. But most of all, be prepared to follow your intuition and trust your feelings, because it is your own, inner ability to heal yourself which will help you.

## Choosing the right therapy: factors to take into consideration

Most forms of complementary medicine work on the basis that if they improve your health, then the individual symptoms will automatically get better. This makes it difficult when it comes to choosing the most appropriate therapy for your particular problem because almost any therapy may relieve almost any disease. This means you need to take a very broad, personal look at the options.

## *Availability*

The therapy should be readily available to you. To take a silly example, you could choose a therapy which is only available in Switzerland and costs thousands of pounds, but it would be a lot simpler if it was available at a reasonable price, close to where you live. So the two key factors are location and cost.

### LOCATION

One of the first steps in choosing the right therapy is to look around and see what is available in your area. Look at the cards and fliers at your local healthfood shop, and the advertisements under 'Health' in your local newspaper. Pick up leaflets from your nearest natural health centre. These will all give you an idea of the kind of therapies which are available in your area.

### COST

Thinking about what you can afford can narrow the choice of what is available in your price range (see the section on 'Money matters', page 242).

The choice of therapy will also depend, at least in part, on whether you are:

- Healthy and want to stay that way, or
- Ill and want to feel well.

## *People who are basically healthy and want to stay that way*

The next question is do you want to do something for yourself, or do you want someone else to do it for you?

If you want to be actively involved and take a do-it-yourself approach then there are plenty of therapies to choose from. Examples include:

- Meditation
- T'ai chi
- Chi gong
- Yoga

- Alexander Technique
- Bates Method of better eyesight
- Diet and nutrition.

It is also a good idea to consider how sociable you feel. Do you relish the idea of going to a class and meeting other people? If so, you might enjoy T'ai chi, Chi gong, or yoga. Or would you prefer to be the centre of attention, in which case you might enjoy the Alexander Technique with its one-to-one tuition.

You may also want to take a look at your whole lifestyle and see how you can make improvements in the way you live your life. Of course you can do this in a fairly random way on your own, but it can be helpful to go to an expert and see a practitioner in a traditional system of medicine, such as Ayurveda, traditional Chinese medicine or naturopathy. Traditional medicine is a useful way of understanding ourselves and our health. Such therapies can diagnose the underlying patterns in your life, the ways you are most likely to lose your balance and fall ill and the ways you can stop that from happening.

If all this sounds like too much like hard work, you may want to try one of the relaxing therapies which will help you to counteract the stresses in your life. Choose from:

- Massage (if you don't mind taking your clothes off)
- Reflexology (where only your feet need to be naked)
- Shiatsu (for massage with your clothes on)
- Healing (which involves keeping your clothes on, and the lightest possible touch – some healers work just away from the skin)
- Zero balancing (you can keep your clothes on, touch is at bone level).

## People who are ill and want to become healthy

Being ill covers a multitude of ailments from a finger ache to a heart attack. Because complementary medicine is based on you rather than your illness, you can narrow the choice by asking questions about the kind of therapy you would feel comfortable with.

## Do I want a therapy that is as much like ordinary medicine as possible?

In other words, would you like to go to a practitioner, be asked a few questions and be given the natural equivalent of ordinary medicine?

If the answer is yes, it would probably be a good idea to choose something like herbal medicine or homeopathy.

## Do you want a therapy that is quite similar to ordinary medicine but where you can talk about your health and your problems?

If the answer is yes, try homeopathy. Homeopaths give you plenty of opportunities to talk about your health and your life.

## Would you rather not have to talk too much, but have someone do something for you?

If the answer is yes, try acupuncture, healing or one of the physical therapies. One of the advantages of acupuncture is that the therapist can find out a lot about you and your health simply by looking at your tongue and feeling your pulses.

Whether or not you choose acupuncture will depend partly on how you feel about needles. The needles that acupuncturists use are really thin and do not feel like injections. But if the idea still makes you squirm, then acupuncture is obviously not for you, try one of the other traditional Chinese medicine therapies such as shiatsu.

## How frightened are you – do you need to have reassurance?

If you have had a heart attack, or if you have suffered from a major illness like cancer, then you may feel that your health has let you down in some way and feel frightened of it happening again. If this is the situation, then acupuncture or any form of traditional Chinese medicine may be worth trying. By looking at your tongue and feeling your pulse, a TCM practitioner can tell what is happening – both with your physical body and with your energy.

## How much of a commitment are you able to make in getting well again?

This is an important question because some forms of therapy rely fairly heavily on you doing something to help yourself. This is particularly true of traditional systems of medicine such as Ayurveda or naturopathy where you may be asked to eat or avoid certain foods and/or practise gentle exercises.

Some people welcome the chance to do something which will help them get better, while others may be too ill or too unwilling to make changes. Homeopathy, healing, acupuncture and herbalism can be helpful if you are unable to do very much to help yourself.

## How much energy do you have?

If you feel wiped out and have very little energy, it would be a good idea to choose a therapy that can help you to build up your energy again.

Choose one of the energy therapies such as homeopathy, healing or acupuncture. Herbal medicine, and nutritional and dietary therapy may also be useful.

## How mobile are you?

If you feel stiff and cannot move around very easily, you may be unwilling to go to one of the physical therapies such as massage, osteopathy, or chiropractic. In fact, these are the very therapies which may be most able to help you. It would certainly be worth going to an osteopath or a chiropractor for an assessment to find out whether they think they can help you.

But if you do not like the thought of having your body touched, or your joints moved, then obviously the physical therapies are not for you and you would be better off with one of the energy medicines or traditional medicines.

## How frail are you?

If you are very frail, it is a good idea to go to one of the gentle energy therapies such as acupuncture, homeopathy or healing. Herbal medicine can also have a strengthening effect.

## WHAT ARE YOUR CIRCUMSTANCES?

Sometimes people live in very difficult circumstances – perhaps on their own, a long way from family and friends, having lost their nearest and dearest. Such difficulties may be caused, or made worse, by the fact that a person lives far away from shops and entertainment.

Some people have a partner who is dying, and find it difficult to cope. Everyone has times when everything seems to get on top of them. It is in just such situations that counselling can be particularly helpful.

## *The nature of the problem*

It is important to begin by thinking about what exactly it is that hurts. Often, it is the problem itself that helps you decide on the best therapy. Examples of this are shown below.

### EMOTIONAL PROBLEMS

If the problem is essentially an emotional one it can help to talk things through, so try one of the talking therapies such as counselling or psychotherapy. But you may also need some extra energy to resolve the cause of the emotional distress, so try one of the energy therapies as well. Healing, homeopathy and Bach flower remedies can help to resolve long standing emotional problems.

Both types of therapy are useful: the talking therapies give you insight, and the energy therapies give you the boost you need to make a change.

### ACHES AND PAINS IN THE BONES OR JOINTS

The most obvious choice in such a situation is for one of the physical therapies such as osteopathy, chiropractic, massage or zero balancing. If you would prefer not to be touched, then try one of the energy therapies or herbal medicine.

### DIGESTIVE PROBLEMS, CONSTIPATION AND DIARRHOEA

Try the traditional medicines such as traditional Chinese medicine, Ayurvedic medicine or naturopathy, as these all address the issue of what you should be eating, and adjust it to your individual needs. If you would prefer not to change your diet, then try kinesiology, herbal medicine or one of the energy therapies.

## HEART AND CIRCULATION PROBLEMS

The therapy you choose will largely depend on how serious the problem is. Obviously varicose veins pose a much less severe problem than heart failure! In the early stages of heart disease it is important to prevent it getting worse, so you need help and support with your lifestyle to help you avoid problems in the future. One of the traditional medicines such as TCM, Ayurvedic medicine or naturopathy would be particularly helpful here. Consider very gentle exercise such as T'ai chi or Chi gong.

If your heart disease is quite severe and you have very little energy, then herbal medicine can be particularly helpful. Also consider one of the energy therapies such as acupuncture, healing or homeopathy.

## CANCER

There are many different therapies that can be useful including:

- Diet and nutrition
- Relaxation and visualisation
- Healing
- Acupuncture/homeopathy
- Herbal medicine

If you have cancer it is a good idea to go to the Bristol Cancer Help Centre, or your local cancer support group for help and advice.

## When did the problem start?

This is a question which is often asked by complementary medicine practitioners, and it can help you to choose the most appropriate therapy for you.

For example, if you became ill:

**After an accident**     Try one of the physical therapies such as chiropractic or osteopathy.

| After a bereavement | Try one of the talking therapies and/or one of the energy therapies. |
| After an infection or virus | Try one of the energy therapies such as homeopathy, acupuncture or healing or a form of traditional medicine such as Ayurveda, traditional Chinese medicine or naturopathy. |

## On death and dying

Dying takes a certain amount of energy as we change from one state of being to another. One of the energy therapies may be helpful as they can often bring peace and serenity to the situation. Spiritual healing is particularly helpful at this time. Counselling and aromatherapy may also help.

### DOES IT HURT?

Complementary medicine can be particularly helpful in easing pain. When the disease is incurable, and all that can be done amounts to little more than relieving the pain, the treatment is known as 'palliative care'.

The best kind of treatment will partly depend on how bad the pain is and whether you are able to help yourself.

Self-help techniques to try include relaxation, visualisation and biofeedback. But if you are in too ill to help yourself, acupuncture, healing, homeopathy or aromatherapy may be helpful.

## Choosing the right therapist: factors to take into consideration

'When the student is ready the teacher appears'. Although this saying applies to students and teachers it is just as appropriate when it comes to finding the right therapist. Your own vital force will attract the therapist you need. In some ways choosing the right therapist is even more important than choosing the right therapy. After all, any therapy is only as good as its practitioner.

## *Logical factors*

There are two types of factor to bear in mind when you are looking for a therapist – the logical and the emotional. First, let us look at the logical factors. You need to find a therapist who is:

- Qualified
- Trained
- Experienced
- Successful.

### QUALIFICATIONS

You need to find a practitioner who is qualified to practice whatever it is they are practising. This means that they should belong to the relevant professional body and have the appropriate qualifications. If you are in doubt about which professional body they should belong to or what qualifications they should have, contact the Institute of Complementary Therapies (address on page 257) which will be able to help.

### TRAINING

Some therapies offer qualifications after a relatively short period of time, while others demand training at degree level or higher.

If the therapist also happens to be a medically trained doctor it is a particularly good idea to find out how long they trained in complementary therapy. Doctors are usually allowed to practise natural therapies after relatively little training compared to their professional colleagues.

Even amongst professional complementary medicine practitioners, the length of time it can take to learn the different therapies varies widely. For example, it is possible to learn massage in 100 hours, although some massage therapists have undergone 1600 hours of training.

The best practitioners never stop learning, so it is a good idea to find out whether they still go on training courses or are developing their practice in some other way (such as through teaching, which is an excellent way to learn).

## EXPERIENCE

The best therapists take good care of themselves and have personal experience in the therapy they practise. For example, if a particular hypnotherapist still smokes, you may not want to go to them to help you give up smoking. On the other hand, you do not want your therapist to be perfect, otherwise how would they be able to empathise with you and understand your problems?

It is a good idea to find out how long the therapist has been practising that particular therapy for. We all learn by our mistakes, and the longer a therapist has been in practice, the more mistakes they will have made and the more they will know. If you are well and just want to stay that way, then experience is not quite so important, but if you are frail, then you need the most experienced practitioner you can find.

This is very important. It is even worth saying again. If you are ill, then you need the most experienced practitioner that you can find. The more frail you are, the more experienced your practitioner needs to be, so that they are able to give you the best possible care.

## SUCCESS

How busy is the therapist you are interested in? This is particularly important in private medicine where you have to pay for your treatment. Generally speaking, the busier the therapist, the more successful they are. If they are successful, then they will probably have helped a lot of people and so they are more likely to be able to help you. There are exceptions to the busy rule. Some excellent practitioners go through quiet patches – or they may have only recently moved into the area, or they may have just come back after having a long period away (for example, on maternity leave).

## Emotional factors

Your therapist has to 'feel' right. We all instinctively know when something or someone is right for us – it is not as dramatic as falling in love, but there are similarities. You should feel better in some way just by knowing that this particular person is going to treat you. Try asking yourself some questions:

- Do you trust this person?
- Do you think that the therapist is genuinely interested in you and your problems?
- Was there any kind of happy coincidence involved in finding them – for example, did several different people recommend the same therapist?

Be prepared to use trial and error before you find the therapist or therapists who you feel happy working with.

## How to find the right practitioner in the private sector

The best way to find the right practitioner is through word of mouth. Ask your friends, ask your acquaintances, ask your hairdresser, dentist, ask anyone you meet – do they know of any good complementary therapists? If you live in a small town, the chances are that there are a few therapists who have excellent reputations – if several people all mention the same therapist, then it is certainly worth finding out more about them.

People who work in healthfood shops tend to know the local practitioners and if you talk to them, they will probably be able to recommend therapists to you. Natural health centres are also good sources of information about local practitioners, but they will tend to recommend the people who work at the centre.

If you have a particular disease, such as cancer or diabetes, there may be a self help group in your area. It is a good idea to go to at least one of their meetings to see whether this is a group of people you want to join up with for mutual support. People in the group may know of local complementary medicine practitioners with experience in treating your particular disease. They may also have tips about what helped them – and what may help you. If there is no local self help group there may be a national organisation which can help. If you have cancer, for example, you may want to contact the Bristol Cancer Help Centre for advice.

If you live in London, or any large city, then you are bound to have a wider choice – sometimes the choice can be too wide, too bewildering, so you may need to go back to basics.

Decide which therapy you are interested in and phone up the professional organisation associated with the therapy. The organisation will be able to recommend someone in your area who is suitably qualified. Ask for as many names as possible. Shop around, if one does not feel right, then try another.

## How to find a therapist

- Word of mouth
- Healthfood shop
- Alternative book shop
- Natural health centre
- Hairdressers and beauty salons
- Patient support groups
- Public libraries
- Local yellow pages and other directories
- Newspapers and magazines
- Doctor's surgery
- Professional organisations

## Money matters

The cost of treatment can vary enormously, depending on all sorts of factors which may have little or nothing to do with the skills of the practitioner. Fees will depend largely on where the therapist practices from. Generally speaking, the grander the premises, the more expensive the fees. Therapists who work from home will have fewer overheads and should charge less than if they are in Harley Street for example. Fees also vary in different parts of the country. Expect to pay less outside London.

Fees will also vary slightly depending on how long the therapist has been practising – you may have to pay more for more experienced practitioners, on the other hand you may not.

Expect to pay a minimum of £20–£30 an hour for most therapies and a minimum of £50 for a first homeopathic consultation which will probably take more than an hour.

When you are thinking about the costs and whether they are worth it, it is important to find out what you are paying for, and how often you may have to pay for it. For example, if you go to a homeopath you may be charged quite a lot of money for the first appointment. But the fee will probably include any medicine and you are unlikely to need another appointment for at least four to six weeks and follow up appointments will probably be cheaper. On the other hand, if you go to an acupuncturist, you may have to go every week for a few weeks and the acupuncturist may suggest that you also take Chinese herbs which will cost a few pounds on top of the fee for the acupuncture treatment.

As a nation, we are not used to paying for medical treatment, so deciding to pay for complementary medicine can be quite a leap. Paying for treatment does have some advantages though. When you are paying for someone's services it 'makes you the boss' which can be very empowering. It puts you in charge of the healing process.

It is important to think about what you can afford in a realistic way. Sometimes the answer is very clear – you may be able to easily afford treatment, or it may be that paying the full cost of treatment is simply out of the question: you cannot afford it and you have no savings. But matters of money are seldom clear cut. Sometimes it is a matter of priority, a priority which only you can decide on. Seeing a complementary therapist can mean making changes in your life – just wanting to feel healthier means that you want to change. Sometimes it is not easy to make changes, which is why answering some of these questions may be more challenging than they first seem.

- Is it more important to spend money on smoking or drinking alcohol than looking after your health?
- Is it more important to have your hair coloured and permed than to look after your health?
- Is it more important to buy treats for the children and grandchildren, or look after your own health?
- Would you rather spend a fortune at the healthfood shop on pills and potions or see an expert who will tell you what you need and what you don't need.
- Is it more important to run a large house or take care of your health? Selling your home and moving to a smaller place is a

difficult decision, but doing so can release a lot of energy as well as money.

You may find it helpful to discuss the issues with a friend, a relative – or even a counsellor. It may be a question of deciding how to spend your money or you may actually be in a situation where you simply cannot afford to pay the full price for complementary medicine. Fortunately there are an increasing number of free and low cost options available.

## Free and low cost treatment

Free and low cost treatment is becoming available to increasing numbers of people as the benefits of complementary medicine come to be recognised. However, the availability of free and low cost treatment is very varied, and depends largely on where you live and what is available locally.

## How to get complementary medicine through your GP

An increasing number of GPs are offering complementary medicine as part of the NHS service.

### Complementary medicine in general practice

A study carried out in 1995 showed that:

- 40 per cent of GP surgeries provided access to some form of complementary medicine
- 21 per cent offered treatment by a member of the primary health care team
- 6 per cent employed an independent complementary therapist
- 25 per cent referred patients to complementary therapists
- 83 per cent of patients did not have to pay for complementary treatment

Source: Thomas, K., Fell, M., Parry, G., Nicholl, J. *National Survey of Access to Complementary Health Care via General Practice*. Medical Care Research Unit, University of Sheffield, August 1995.

There has been a huge shift in the way doctors view complementary medicine. In the early 1960s, doctors could be struck off the register for committing any of the three A's: alcholism, advertising and association. 'Association' included associating with 'undesirables' such as alternative health practitioners! Talking to complementary therapists let alone referring patients to them was forbidden.

Forty years later, times have changed and increasing numbers of doctors are welcoming complementary medicine with open arms. According to the latest survey, more than three quarters of GPs want acupuncture to be available on the NHS. (See *Acupuncture: Efficacy and Practice*, British Medical Association Board of Science and Education, Harwood Academic, 2000).

If you want any form of complementary medicine on the NHS all you can really do is ask. Whether or not you get it will largely depend on the facilities that are available in your area and how sympathetic your GP is to the idea. At the Glastonbury Health Centre, it is possible to get acupuncture, osteopathy, massage and herbalism for the price of an NHS prescription, but the centre has had to set up a charity to pay for the service. Other doctors' surgeries pay for the services of a complementary medicine practitioner as part of their budget.

- If you are interested in homeopathy you can ask your GP to refer you to the nearest homeopathic hospital for treatment.
- If you are interested in Ayurvedic medicine you can ask your GP to refer you to the new free Ayurvedic hospital in London.
- If you have a bad back, you can ask your GP to refer you to an osteopath or a chiropractor as these therapies are now widely recognised as being good for back pain. In 1996, the Royal College of General Practitioners issued guidelines for GPs which recommend manipulative treatment within the first six weeks for patients with low back pain.

Your GP is the gatekeeper to the services which are available on the NHS. Some GPs go out of their way to find ways of providing complementary medicine for their patients. Your GP is most likely to be sympathetic if:

- Normal investigations cannot find the reason for your symptoms.
- Conventional treatment has not worked.
- Conventional treatment has caused side effects.
- You are newly diagnosed with a serious complaint that is unlikely to respond to conventional treatment.

If your GP is unsympathetic to complementary medicine, you may want to consider changing your GP.

## Physiotherapy

Physiotherapists are trained to do massage and offer advice on diet, exercise and lifestyles – they can be an excellent starting point if you want to take a more natural approach to your healthcare within the NHS framework.

## How to get low cost complementary medicine in the private sector

- Most complementary medicine practitioners offer concessions to people who cannot afford the full fee – ask if the practitioner offers treatment at reduced cost. This is sometimes called a sliding scale.
- Some natural health centres offer therapies on a donation basis, so ask your local natural health centre what they offer.
- Self help groups may know of practitioners in the area who offer low cost treatment.
- If you live in an area where there is a school of complementary medicine, there may be a free or low cost students clinic.

# Choosing a respectable therapy

Some therapies were given the seal of respectability by the recent House of Lords Select Committee on Science and Technology. In their report on Complementary and Alternative Medicine, they identified three types of therapy:

**Group 1:** (Also known as 'The Big Five'). These are the most respectable therapies: osteopathy, chiropractic, acupuncture, herbal medicine and homeopathy. These were chosen because they were well organised and well researched or likely to respond well to research. Osteopathy and chiropractic are already regulated by Acts of Parliament, and the other therapies in this section may also become regulated. Therapists who practice Group 1 therapies diagnose symptoms as well as provide treatment.

**Group 2:** These therapies most clearly complement conventional medicine and some are already used in the NHS, especially among the terminally ill. Therapists in this group will sometimes refer you to your own GP as they do not offer diagnosis. This group includes aromatherapy, the Alexander Technique, body work therapies including massage, counselling, stress therapy, hypnotherapy, reflexology, shiatsu, meditation and healing.

**Group 3:** These therapies are the outsiders which are unlikely to attract research funding or be included within the NHS. Strangely enough this group includes traditional therapies such as traditional Chinese medicine, even though acupuncture (part of TCM) was given the Group 1 seal of approval. Kinesiology is also in Group 3, even though it is often used by chiropractors who are also included under Group 1. Group 3 also includes Ayurvedic medicine, crystal therapy, iridology, radionics and dowsing.

Reference: *Complementary and Alternative Medicine*, House of Lords Select Committee on Science and Technology, 1999–2000, The Stationery Office.

# A personal note to conclude

While I have been writing this book I have been struck by the number of therapies that I have used myself – particularly in the past two years since I had a heart attack. Looking at the list it almost reads like the contents page of this book! Different therapies have helped me in different ways at different stages of my recovery.

When I had my heart attack I was given spiritual healing in the intensive care unit of the local hospital. When I went onto the general ward I was given *The Heart Manual* to work through which told me what I could do to help myself with diet, exercises and relaxation. The staff nurse from the casualty ward lent me a relaxation tape. The physiotherapist I worked with did not just give me exercises to do, she also helped me to regain my confidence and gave me all sorts of holistic advice and encouragement.

When I got home I had regular healing from spiritual healers. The heart support group at the local hospital was helpful and I was fortunate because I also had on-going support from the physiotherapist.

I had counselling to help me to rebuild my life. I was offered cognitive counselling from my GP's surgery, but chose a more holistic approach from a private counsellor who several friends had recommended.

I had homeopathy which was dramatically helpful when I had pneumonia and the doctor's antibiotics were not shifting it.

I have also had acupuncture and Chinese herbs which have not only helped my recovery, but my acupuncturist was able to give me valuable feedback on how my health has been progressing. I have just started doing yoga and am really enjoying it.

Complementary medicine has certainly helped me to feel well again in body, mind, emotions and spirit – and I'm sure it will help you to do so too.

# Bibliography

Achterberg, J. (1985) *Imagery and Healing*. Shambhala Press.

Ader, R., Fellen, D., Cohen, N. (1990) *Psychoneuroimmunology* (2nd edition). Academic Press.

Alexander, F.M. (Reissued 1986) *The Use of the Self*. Gollancz.

Bates, W.H. (1919: re-issued 2000) *Better Eyesight without Glasses*. Thorsons.

Bird, L. (1999) *The Fundamental Facts*. The Mental Health Foundation.

Borrill, J. *All about Depression*. The Mental Health Foundation.

BMA Board of Science and Education (2000) *Acupuncture: Efficacy and Practice*. Harwood Academic.

Chappell, P., Andrews, D. (1996) *Healing with Homeopathy*. Gill & Macmillan.

Charlton, J., Murphy, M. (1995) *The Health of Adult Britain 1841–1994*. Office for National Statistics, The Stationery Office.

Ch'ing, C.M. (1991) *T'ai Chi Ch'uan*. North Atlantic Books.

Chopra, D. (1993) *Ageless Body, Timeless Mind*. Rider.

Clark, S. (2000) 'Zero balancing – a therapy to harmonise mind and body'. *The Times*, September 28.

Conable, B., Conable, W. (1992) *How to Learn the Alexander Technique – A Manual for Students*. Andover Road Publishers.

D'Adamo, P., Whitney, C. (1998) *The Eat Right Diet*. Century.

Daniel, R. (2000) *Healing Foods*. Thorsons.

Daniel, R. (2000) *Living with Cancer*. Robinson.

Davis, P. (1995) *Aromatherapy An A–Z* (revised edition). Daniel.

Department of Health (1991) *Dietary Reference Values for Food Energy and Nutrients for the United Kingdom*. Report of the Panel on Dietary Reference Values. HMSO.

Dougans, I., Ellis, S. (1992) *The Art of Reflexology*. Element books.

Downing, G. (1989) *The Massage Book*. Arkana.

Dziemidko, H. (1999) *The Complete Book of Energy Medicine*. Gaia.

Endacott, M. (1997) *Encyclopaedia of Complementary Medicine*. Grange Books.

Gerzon, M. (1996) *Listening to Midlife – Turning your Crisis into a Quest*. Shambhala Press.

Grant, D., Joice, J. (1984) *Food Combining for Health*. Thorsons.

Gross, R. *et al.* (1978) 'Aging: Real and Imaginary' in *New Old: Struggling for Decent Ageing*. Anchor.

Hamwee, J. (2000) *Zero Balancing*. Frances Lincoln.

Herzberg, E.I. (1998) *Spiritual Healing – A Patient's Guide*. Daniel.

Hilgard, E.R. (1965) *Hypnotic Sensibility*. Harcourt Brace.

Holdway, A (1995) *Kinesiology*. Element Books.

House of Lords Select Committee on Science and Technology (2000) *Complementary and Alternative Medicine*. The Stationery Office.

Huxley, A. (1941) *The Art of Seeing*. Chatto & Windus.

Kenton, L. (1994) *New Raw Energy*. Vermilion.

Kenton, L. (1995) *Ageless Ageing*; 2nd edition. Vermilion.

Kenton, L. (1999) *Raw Energy Food Combining Diet*. Ebury Press.

Kielczynski, W. (1997) Osteoarthritis clinical outcomes after uniform long term treatment. *European Journal of Herbal Medicine*, vol 3, no 2 (Autumn).

Kinsella, K., Gist, Y.J. (1998) *International Brief: Gender and Aging, Mortality and Health*. International Programs Center, US Department of Commerce Economics and Statistics, Administration Bureau of the Census, October 1998.

Kirkwood, T. (1999) *Time of Our Lives: The Science of Human Aging*. Phoenix Publishers.

Kübler-Ross, E. (1970) *On Death and Dying*. Tavistock Publications.

Kyle, L. (1998/9) 'Aromatherapy for elder care'. *International Journal of Aromatherapy*, vol 9, no 4.

La Tourelle, M., Courtnay, A. (1992) *Thorsons Introductory Guide to Kinesiology*. Thorsons.

Le Tissier, J. (1992) *Food Combining for Vegetarians*. Thorsons.

Lorius, C. (2001) *Homeopathy for the Soul*. Thorsons.

MacBeth, J. (1981) *Sun Over Mountain*. Gateway.

MacBeth, J. (1990) *Moon Over Water*. Gateway.

Mansfield, P. (1995) *The Bates Method*. Vermilion.

McCay, C. (1950) 'Clinical aspects of ageing and the effect of diet upon ageing. In *Cowdry's Problems of Ageing* (3rd edition). Williams & Williams Co.

Mental Health Foundation (Updated regularly) *Someone to Talk to Directory*. Published on the Internet and available at www.mental-health.org.uk.

Mental Health Foundation Survey (1997) *Knowing Our Own Minds*. Mental Health Foundation.

Mitchell, S (1979) *Naturopathy*. Blackwell.

Moody, H.R. (1998) *Ageing Concepts and Controversies.*, Pine Forge Press.

Morrison, J. (1995) *The Book of Ayurveda*. Gaia.

Pert, C. (1997) *Molecules of Emotion*. Simon & Schuster

Pitchford, P. (1996) *Healing with Whole Foods*. North Atlantic Books.

Price, S., Price, L. (1995) *Aromatherapy for Health Professionals*. Churchill Livingstone.

Ross, M.H. *et al.* (1972) 'Length of life and caloric intake'. *American Journal of Clinical Nutrition*, vol 25 (August).

Sanders, P. (1998) *First Steps in Counselling*. PCCS Books.

Schneider, M. (1997) *Meir Schneider's Miracle Eyesight Method: The Natural Way to Heal and Improve your Vision.* Sounds True Audiocassette.

Scrutton, S. (1995) *Bereavement and Grief: Supporting Older People Through Loss.* Edward Arnold and Age Concern.

Sen, J. (1996) *The Healing Foods Cookbook.* Thorsons.

Smith, F. (1986) *Inner Bridges.* Humanics New Age.

Stevens, C. (1987) *Alternative Health: Alexander Technique.* Optima.

Thomas, K., Fell, M., Parry, G., Nicholl, J. (1995) *National Survey of Access to Complementary Health Care via General Practice.* Medical Care Research Unit, University of Sheffield.

Tschudin, V. (1999) *Counselling and Older People: An introductory guide.* Age Concern Books.

Valnet, J. (1980) *The Practice of Aromatherapy.* Daniel.

Warrior, G., Gunawar, D. (1997) *The Complete Illustrated Guide to Ayurveda.* Element.

Weeks. D., James, J. (1998) *Superyoung.* Hodder & Stoughton.

# Useful addresses

**Academy of Oriental Medicine**
28 Wood Street
Lytham St Annes
Lancashire SY8 1QR
Tel: 01253 728035

**Acupuncture Association of Chartered Physiotherapists**
The Mere Complementary Practice
Castle Street
Mere
Wiltshire BA12 6JE
Tel: 01747 861151

**Aromatherapy Organisations Council**
PO Box 19834
London SE25 6WF
Tel: 020 8251 7912
Website: www.aoc.uk.org

**Ayurvedic Charitable Hospital**
81 Wimpole Street
London W1M 7DB
Tel: 020 7224 6070
Email: acgb@cs.com

**Ayurvedic Company of Great Britain**
50 Penywern Road
London SW5 9SX
Tel: 020 7370 2255
*For a list of qualified practitioners.*

**Dr Edward Bach Centre**
Mount Vernon
Bakers Lane
Sotwell
Oxfordshire OX10 0PZ
Tel: 01491 834678

**Bates Association for Vision Education**
PO Box 25
Shoreham-by-Sea
West Sussex BN43 6ZF
Tel: 01273 422090
Email: bave@seeing.org
Website: www.seeing.org

**British Academy of Western Acupuncture**
12 Poulton Green Close
Spital
Wirral CH63 9FS
Tel: 0151 343 9168

**British Acupuncture Council**
63 Jeddo Road
London W12 9HQ
Tel: 020 8735 0400

**British Association for Applied Chiropractic**
The Old Post Office
Cherry Street
Stratton Audley
Bicester
Oxfordshire OX6 9BA
Tel: 01869 277111

**British Association for Counselling**
37A Sheep Street
Rugby
Warwickshire CV21 3BX
Tel: 01788 578328
Website: www.counselling.co.uk
*Gives information on counselling services nationwide.*

**British Association of Nutritional Therapists**
27 Old Gloucester Street
London WC1N 3XX
Tel: 0870 606 1284
*260 names currently on the register. A minimum of two years training is needed.*

**British Chiropractic Association**
29 Whitley Street
Reading
Berkshire RG2 0EG
Tel: 0118 950 5950
Website: www.chiropractic-uk.co.uk

**British Massage Therapy Council**
17 Rymers Lane
Oxford OX4 4JU
Tel: 01865 774123

**British Medical Acupuncture Society**
Royal London Homeopathic Hospital
60 Great Ormond Street
London WC1N 3HR
Tel: 020 7278 1615

**British Naturopathic Association**
Goswell House
2 Goswell Road
Street
Somerset BA16 0JG
Tel: 01458 840072
Website: www.naturopathy.org.uk

**British Rebirth Society**
Margot Messenger – General Secretary
5 Durham House
Fieldway Crescent
London N5 1AG

**British Reflexology Association**
Monks Orchard
Whitbourne
Worcester
WR6 5RB
Tel: 01886 821207
Fax: 01886 822017
Website: www.britreflex.co.uk

**Centre for Transpersonal Psychology**
86A Marylebone High Street
London W1N 3DE
Tel: 020 7935 7350

**Chiropractic Patients Association**
8 Centre One
Lysander Way
Old Sarum Park
Salisbury
Wiltshire SP4 6BU
Tel: 01722 415027

**Co-Counselling International**
c/o Westerly
Prestwick Lane
Chiddingfold
Surrey GU8 4XW

**Confederation of Healing Organisations**
PO Box 624
Hemel Hempstead
Hertfordshire HP3 0QF
Tel: 01442 244296

**Cruse Bereavement Care**
126 Sheen Road
Richmond
Surrey TW9 1UR
Tel: 020 8940 4818
*Provides comfort in bereavement, and can put you in touch with people in your area.*

**Doctor–Healer Network**
27 Montefiore Court
Stamford Hill
London N16 5TY
Tel: 020 8800 3569

**Faculty of Homeopaths**
15 Clerkenwell Close
London EC1R 0AA
Tel: 020 7566 7810

**General Council and Register of Naturopaths**
Goswell House
2 Goswell Road
Street
Somerset BA16 0JG
Tel: 01458 840072
Website: www.naturopathy.org.uk

**General Osteopathic Council**
Osteopathy House
176 Tower Bridge Road
London SE1 3LU
Tel: 020 7357 6655
Website: www.osteopathy.org.uk

**Healing Foundation**
Half Acre House
Upper Battlefield
Shrewsbury
Shropshire SY4 4AA
Tel: 01939 210980

**Institute of Complementary Therapies**
PO Box 194
London SE16 7QZ
Tel: 020 7237 5165 (10–3pm)
Website: www.icmedicine.co.uk

**Kinesiology Federation**
PO Box 17153
Edinburgh EH11 3WQ
Tel: 08700 113545
Email: kfadmin@kinesiologyfederation.org
Website: www.kinesiologyfederation.org

**McTimoney Chiropractic Association**
21 High Street
Eynsham
Oxfordshire OX8 1HE
Tel: 01865 880974
Website: www.McTimoney-chiropractic.org

**Mental Health Foundation**
20–21 Cornwall Terrace
London Nw1 4QL
Tel: 020 7535 7400
Email: mhf@mentalhealth.org.uk
Website: www.mentalhealth.org.uk

**Metamorphic Association**
67 Ritherdon Road
London SW17 8QE
Tel: 020 8672 5951

**MIND**
Granta House
15-19 Broadway
London E15 4BQ
Tel: 020 8519 2122
*Provides information, support and publications about all aspects of mental illness, depression etc.*

**National Association of Bereavement Services**
29 Norton Folgate
London E1 6DB
Tel: 020 7247 0617
*Provides a directory database of local and national services. Also runs a referral help line manned by trained bereavement counsellors who give information, advice and referral to a caller's nearest and most appropriate service.*

**National Federation of Spiritual Healers**
The Old Manor Farm Studio
Church Street
Sunbury-on-Thames
Middlesex TW16 6RG
Tel: 01932 783164
*(For information about training to be a healer)*
Tel: 09068 616080 (premium rate line)
*(If you want to contact local healers)*

**National Institute of Medical Herbalists**
56 Longbrook Street
Exeter EX4 4AH
Tel: 01392 426022

**Reiki Association**
Cornbrook Bridge House
Clee Hill
Ludlow SY 8QQ
Tel: 07970 207257
Website: www.reikiassociation.org.uk

**Relate**
Herbert Gray College
Little Church Street
Rugby
Warwickshire CV21 3AP
Tel: 01788 573241/560811
*Counselling and help with difficult relationships; many local branches*

**Scottish Chiropractic Association**
30 Roseburn Place
Edinburgh EH12 5NX
Tel: 0131 346 7500

**Shiatsu Society**
Eastlands Court
St Peters Road
Rugby CV21 3QP
Tel: 01788 555051
Email: admin@shiatsu.org
Website: www.shiatsu.org

**UK Council for Psychotherapy**
167-169 Great Portland Street
London WC1N 5FB
Tel: 020 7436 3002
Website: www.psychotherapy.org.uk

**ZBA UK**
10 Victoria Grove
Bridport
Dorset DT6 3AA
Tel: 01308 420007
Website: www.zerobalancing.com

# About Age Concern

*Know Your Complementary Therapies* is one of a wide range of publications produced by Age Concern England, the National Council on Ageing. Age Concern works on behalf of all older people and believes later life should be fulfilling and enjoyable. For too many this is impossible. As the leading charitable movement in the UK concerned with ageing and older people, Age Concern finds effective ways to change that situation.

Where possible, we enable older people to solve problems themselves, providing as much or as little support as they need. A network of local Age Concerns, supported by 250,000 volunteers, provides community-based services such as lunch clubs, day centres and home visiting.

Nationally, we take a lead role in campaigning, parliamentary work, policy analysis, research, specialist information and advice provision, and publishing. Innovative programmes promote healthier lifestyles and provide older people with opportunities to give the experience of a lifetime back to their communities.

Age Concern is dependent on donations, covenants and legacies.

**Age Concern England**
1268 London Road
London SW16 4ER
Tel: 020 8765 7200
Fax: 020 8765 7211

**Age Concern Cymru**
4th Floor
1 Cathedral Road
Cardiff CF1 9SD
Tel: 029 2037 1566
Fax: 029 2039 9562

**Age Concern Scotland**
113 Rose Street
Edinburgh EH2 3DT
Tel: 0131 220 3345
Fax: 0131 220 2779

**Age Concern Northern Ireland**
3 Lower Crescent
Belfast BT7 1NR
Tel: 028 9024 5729
Fax: 028 9023 5497

# Publications from Age Concern Books

Gardening in Retirement

*Bernard Salt*

*Gardening in Retirement* is a new and refreshing approach to gardening, aimed specifically at retired people. It is a book for the fit and active looking for a challenge, but it also contains information useful for those who experience difficulties with everyday tasks. The book:

- contains numerous ideas and tips on making most jobs easier
- covers both organic and conventional approaches to gardening
- contains over 300 colour photographs

Subjects covered include patios, lawns, borders, greenhouses, trees, fruit and vegetables. Safety, recycling, care of wildlife and the environment are also emphasised. Highly practical, the book has something to offer everyone – from those who want to spend happy hours pursuing gardening as a hobby to others who want an easy-to-maintain yet attractive garden.

£12.99   0-86242-311-2

**Know Your Medicines**

*Pat Blair*

This handy guide answers many of the common questions that older people – and those who care for them – often have about the medicines they use and how they work. The text stresses safety throughout, and covers:

- what medicines actually do
- using medicines more effectively
- getting advice and asking questions
- taking your medicine
- medicines and your body systems
- common ailments

There is also information about the dosage and strength, brands, storage and disposal, and an index to help look up medicines that are prescribed or bought over the counter.

£7.99   0-86242-226-4

**Your Rights**
**A guide to money benefits for older people**

*Sally West*

A highly acclaimed annual guide to the State benefits available to older people. Contains information on changes to benefits for people widowed under pension age; Incapacity Benefit; Income Support and the Social Fund; housing and council tax benefits and Retirement Pensions, among other matters, and includes advice on how to claim them.

**Your Taxes and Savings**
**A guide for older people**

*Sally West and the Money Management Council*

Explains how the tax system affects older people over retirement age, including how to avoid paying more than necessary. The wide range of investment opportunities available to older people wishing to make their money work harder are also examined, together with advice on building an investment portfolio, guidance on protection for investors and debt management.

For more information please contact Age Concern Books in Devon.

---

If you would like to order any of these titles, please write to the address below, enclosing a cheque or money order for the appropriate amount (plus £1.95 p&p) made payable to Age Concern England. Credit card orders may be made on 0870 44 22 044 (for individuals); or 0870 44 22 120 (AC federation, other organisations and institutions). Fax: 01626 323318

**Age Concern Books**
PO Box 232
Newton Abbot
Devon TQ12 4XQ

# Age Concern Information Line/Factsheets subscription

Age Concern produces 44 comprehensive factsheets designed to answer many of the questions older people (or those advising them) may have. These include money and benefits, health, community care, leisure and education, and housing. For up to five free factsheets, telephone 0800 00 99 66 (7am–7pm, seven days a week, every day of the year). Alternatively you may prefer to write to Age Concern, FREEPOST (SWB 30375), ASHBURTON, Devon TQ13 7ZZ.

For professionals working with older people, the factsheets are available on an annual subscription service, which includes updates throughout the year. For further details and costs of the subscription, please write to Age Concern at the above Freepost address.

# Index